Caribbean Herbs
for Diabetes Management

Caribbean Herbs
for Diabetes Management:
Fact or Fiction?

Henry I. C. Lowe ▪ Errol Y. St. A. Morrison
Perceval S. Bahado-Singh ▪ Cliff K. Riley

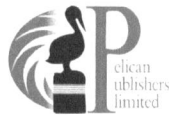

PELICAN PUBLISHERS LIMITED
Kingston, Jamaica W.I.

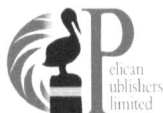

First published in Jamaica, 2012 by Pelican Publishers Limited

44 Lady Musgrave Road
Kingston 10 Jamaica, W.I.
Tel: (876) 978-8377 Fax: (876) 978-0048
Email: pelicanpublishers@gmail.com
Website: www.pelicanpubja.com

© 2012, Henry I.C. Lowe, Errol Y. St. A. Morrison, Perceval S. Bahado-Singh, Cliff K. Riley

ISBN 978-976-8240-01-9

Cover design by Pelican Publishers Limited

Printed in Jamaica by MAPCO Printers Limited.

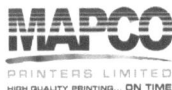

Dedication

To all those who are afflicted with diabetes

Table of Contents

Foreword

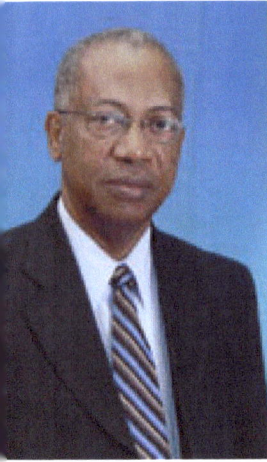

Professor Winston Davidson

The practice of medicine in the twenty-first century requires the development of the skill of health information management in order to cope with the current explosion in the quantity of health information and the diversity of its quality represented by wider varieties of formats and scientific credence. This feature has sometimes been referred to as "information overload" but there is no excuse whatsoever for any practitioner to lack the capacity to manage this situation in such a way that the patients are enabled to make an informed choice irrespective of the nature of their illness or condition.

What has caused this rapid growth and dissemination of this vast volume and varied quality of health information in the public space?

Much of this information is derived from the rapid conversion of voice, video and data to an all-digital format which has led to the access of vast volumes of health information on the internet and the ubiquitous mobile telephone network platforms made available to patients and practitioners in the local public and global spaces. Some of this information is derived from evidence based sources, others from traditional cultural sources while others are mere fabrications developed by charlatans.

The practice of medicine in the twenty-first century demands that all practitioners are not only able to identify health information which is credible but must also be able to properly manage health information from all available sources and to disseminate this credible information to patients in a user friendly format.

This book produced by authors who are world experts in their field satisfies the criteria and features which I have described.

The authors of this book could not have produced a more relevant publication, because it seeks, in the organization of its content, to distinguish between the different qualitative and quantitative levels of scientific evidence necessary to differentiate between conventional medicine, traditional, herbal and ethno medicine, nutraceuticals and pharmaceuticals in the management of one of the most epidemiologically significant diseases in Jamaica and the Caribbean- "Diabetes Mellitus".

There is no publication in the Caribbean which seeks to inform practitioners or patients along these lines.

The authors of this book report that the prevalence of diabetes among persons 25–74 years old in Jamaica is estimated to be between 12 % and 16 % (Wilks et al, 1999; Cooper et al, 1997; Ragoobirsingh et al, 1995). In Latin America and the Caribbean, the highest prevalence rate was registered in Jamaica (17.9 %), and the lowest in Cuba with 11.8 %. This data demonstrates the importance of diabetes as one of the most important epidemiologic challenges in Jamaica and the Caribbean

The management of diabetes mellitus in Jamaica and Caribbean societies has always posed a challenge for practitioners as there is always competition and sometimes contradictions between the use of the prescription of conventional medical treatment by the physician and the patient's concomitant use of traditional, herbal and ethno-medicines derived from traditional folklore sources.

This is the first book published in the Caribbean of credible scientific rigour which attempts successfully to bridge that gap.

What is particularly useful is the fact that the book gives a peer reviewed update of the conventional contemporary treatment of diabetes mellitus in chapters 1 and 2 and in the process it lays out the facts in an easily read format. This feature presents a convenient source of information not only for practitioners but also for patients who wish to inform themselves about their illness from a rigorously credible source. This feature is of immense value to all practitioners of contemporary scientific medicine where patient education for chronic diseases such as diabetes mellitus is a very important component of the treatment regime.

In chapter 3 of the book it has identified plants used in diabetes management to which it attaches the label of "scientifically validated" plants. This chapter is of particular interest as it documents for practitioners, a credible source of information of the local plants which have been used in traditional medicine competing from time to time with conventional pharmaceuticals.

In chapter 4 the book identifies plants suspected to have anti-diabetic properties based on folklore. The importance of this information is of immense value to practitioners not only for the convenience of the source of data but more so as a part of the reference for further work in evaluating clinical outcomes and therefore practitioners may be able to use case studies to enrich the body of knowledge and literature in the management of diabetes mellitus in our unique environments.

The book ends in chapter 5 with suggestions and recommendations on the way forward presenting a vision of the real possibilities for development.

In the final analysis this publication may justifiably be represented as a genuine practitioner's manual as it assists practitioners in addressing challenges in the management of information in the treatment of diabetes mellitus at the level of the communities. The book therefore bridges the knowledge gap between general practice and community health and wellness in Jamaica and presents a vision and framework for future development.

It is therefore a must read and a reference manual for all practitioners who wish to remain relevant and keep abreast of the rapid changes in the vast array of the new emerging health and medical therapeutic industries.

Congratulations to the authors whose efforts must be recognized as being a useful contribution to the management of diabetes mellitus at the level of the practitioner, the patient and the community.

Prof. Winston G. Mendes Davidson, MD, DTM & H (Liverpool)
Head, School of Public Health and Health Technology

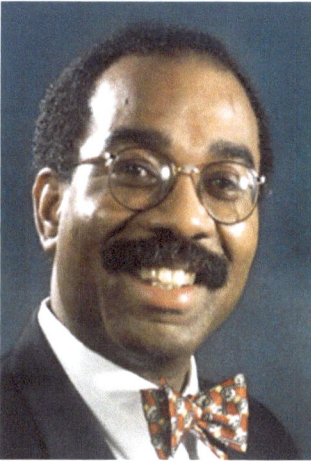

Preface
Professor E. Albert Reece

Diabetes, which was once largely a developed country disease, is now one of the greatest contributors to the global burden of disease, according to the World Health Organization (WHO). WHO estimates that almost 350 million people worldwide currently have diabetes, and, without aggressive intervention, this number is expected to double by the year 2030.

Modern technologies and drugs for monitoring and managing hyperglycemia have made diabetes a very manageable chronic disease, and in the first part of this book, *Caribbean Herbs for Diabetes Management: Fact or Fiction*, the authors provide an excellent and comprehensive discussion of the state of the art of modern glucose detection and control techniques and their potential complications. This is followed by a section on the contribution of nutritional approaches to diabetes management as well as other experimental non-pharmaceutical approaches to diabetes control.

However, many diabetic patients in the developing world cannot afford these modern medicines and technologies, and, thus, may rely on traditional healers or herbal remedies to manage their condition. Thus, the latter part of this book, *Caribbean Herbs for Diabetes Management: Fact or Fiction*, focuses on the most widely used Caribbean plants and folk remedies for diabetes management. The authors provide an excellent discussion of those plants or herbs for which there is some scientific evidence of glucose lowering action, including pictures of the plants, known active ingredients, proposed mechanism of action, and potential toxicities, if known.

However, as the authors point out in their introduction, patients or practitioners who rely on herbs or nutritional approaches alone to manage diabetes do so at their own peril. Indeed, the authorswarnthat"thereisnoclinicalevidencethatconventional therapy for diabetes can be substituted, replaced, or ignored." So, to date, effective herbal remedies for diabetes remain elusive, at best. At worst, they can be potentially dangerous. Thus, the current research on the value of herbs and plant extracts is inconclusive regarding their value for managing diabetes. No human clinical trials, which are the "gold standard" for demonstrating the safety and effectiveness of any therapy, have been performed on herbal remedies in diabetic patients, meaning they cannot currently be recommended as either a substitute or an adjunctive therapy for managing diabetes.

Caribbean Herbs for Diabetes Management: Fact or Fiction? is a valuable primer for anyone wishing to understand diabetes and its consequences as well as those therapies that have been scientifically proven to be effective for its management. It also is an extremely valuable reference manual for those interested in the state of the science of nutritional approaches for managing diabetes. Further research is urgently needed in this area not only to protect diabetic patients from potentially worthless or toxic folk remedies but also to allow us to someday incorporate patients' cultural preferences into their diabetes management plans.

E. Albert Reece, MD, PhD, MBA
Vice President for Medical Affairs, University of Maryland
John Z. and Akiko K. Bowers Distinguished Professor and
Dean, University of Maryland School of Medicine

Acknowledgements

The authors are extremely grateful to all those persons who contributed their time and dedication to work on this very resourceful book. Special thanks to Ms. Shelly McFarlane, Project Manager, North America and Caribbean Region, International Diabetes Federation for her expert review and comments. We are particularly grateful to Mrs Janet Lowe for proof reading the book. We also wish to extend our heartfelt gratitude to Dr. Charah Watson, Ms. Nikeisha Lee, Ms. Shelly-Ann Powell, Ms. Chenee Davis and Ms. Latoya Aquart for their valuable contributions.

Overview

The International Diabetes Federation (IDF) estimates that over 366 million people currently live with diabetes globally. This accounts for 8.3% of the adult population and is projected to increase to near 552 million by 2030. Interestingly, over 80% of persons living with diabetes are from developing countries. In 2001, the prevalence of diabetes mellitus in the English speaking Caribbean ranged from 12.6%–16.4%, with Jamaica (approximately 400,000 cases) and Trinidad and Tobago (approximately 145,000 cases) having the largest number of cases (Figure 1). In 2011, the IDF estimated that 1 in every 10 adults in the North America and Caribbean region has diabetes mellitus (IDF, 2011). The increasing prevalence of diabetes mellitus and associated complications presents significant socio-economic, medical and scientific concerns and challenges. Additionally, the cause "etiology" and nature "pathophysiology" of the disease are markedly different among patients and therefore dictates different prevention strategies, diagnostic screening and treatment methods.

While not much scientific research has been done on alternative management strategies for the disease, traditional herbal concoctions have been used widely in many cultures despite the significant growth in modern pharmaceuticals to treat the disease. Currently, several such traditional remedies continue to play a significant role in the prevention and management of diabetes mellitus in Jamaica and the Caribbean. Research carried out by several local and regional institutions have revealed that a large number of Caribbean plants possess significant activity against hyperglycemia. Examples include Bixa orellana (annatto), Capsicum frutescens (bird pepper), Dioscorea polygonoides (bitter yam). However, most of these scientific breakthroughs have never been commercialized towards the development of nutraceuticals or pharmaceutical products and remain only in the scientific literature.

As such, the authors have carried out an extensive evaluation of the existing scientific literature and have compiled the findings on the eight most widely studied plants with glucose lowering (hypoglycemic) properties along with those without the rigorous scientific support but are still widely used traditionally to prevent or treat diabetes mellitus. We anticipate that this book will serve as a reference to clinicians, scientists and other interest groups to expand on the usefulness and engage in development of novel drugs for the management of diabetes mellitus. Additionally, further research and clinical studies can lead to identification of the extract's safety, effective dosage and drug efficacy. In addition, researchers may utilize this database to investigate those plants with little or no scientific validation for use in the treatment and prevention of diabetes mellitus.

Ethnomedicines/Traditional Medicine

Traditional remedies are widely used in the diagnosis, prevention, treatment and management of a wide-ranging list of diseases and ailments. Persons who use traditional remedies are influenced by numerous factors which have led to their widespread and increasing appeal throughout the Caribbean and globally. Some of the reasons for using traditional medicines include; affordability, cultural practices and thinking and less dependence on conventional medicines.

Despite this and regardless of why an individual uses these forms of remedies, traditional medicines/ethnomedicines provide an essential health care service to persons both with and without financial access to conventional medicine. The use of traditional therapies has demonstrated efficacy and usefulness in areas such as mental health, disease prevention, treatment of non-communicable diseases for example diabetes, and improvement of the quality of life of persons living with diabetes and other chronic diseases. They have also shown great potential to meet a broad spectrum of health care needs. Notwithstanding, additional research, adequate clinical trials, and scientific evaluations are needed.

Recognizing the widespread use of ethnomedicines and the tremendous expansion of international markets for herbal products, it is all the more important to ensure that the health care provided by such plant remedies are safe and reliable; that standards for the safety, efficacy; and quality control of herbal products and therapies are established and strictly adhered to; that researchers and clinicians have the required qualifications; and that all the scientific claims made for products (nutraceuticals or pharmaceuticals) and legal regulations are valid. These issues have become important concerns for both health authorities and the public.

In the Caribbean, ethnomedicines have been used on a wide scale basis for the treatment and management of diabetes. There are numerous plants that are used in different Caribbean countries; some have been investigated and proven by scientists to have anti-diabetic properties whilst others are used based on folkloric use.

However, it is very important to note that even though some medicinal plants may be reported to have some positive effect, it is crucial that we the authors strongly emphasize that "Herbal Therapy" should not be used as a substitute for conventional therapy. In addition, there is "no clinical evidence" that conventional therapy can be substituted, replaced or ignored in the treatment of diabetes.

1

Overview of Diabetes Mellitus

What is Diabetes Mellitus?

Diabetes mellitus, commonly referred to as "sugar", is a disease wherein the glucose in the blood stream is not readily absorbed into the body tissues. Diabetes mellitus may result from the defects in insulin secretion, deficient action of insulin on target tissue (adipose tissue and muscle cells), or complete lack of insulin (Alberti et al, 1999). The chronic hyperglycemia of diabetes mellitus is associated with long-term damage, abnormal function and failure of various organs especially the eyes, kidneys, heart and blood vessels (Mayfield, 1998; Kikkawa, 2000). Those affected may also develop nerve damage (peripheral neuropathy) with the risk of foot ulcers, amputations, and damaged joints as well as other types of nerve damage internally (autonomic neuropathy) causing stomach, and sex organ malfunction.

The vast majority of diabetes mellitus cases fall into two broad categories and are given the names descriptive of their clinical presentation: Type 1 (previously referred to as Insulin-dependent diabetes mellitus: IDDM or juvenile onset diabetes mellitus) and type 2 (previously referred to as non-insulin-dependent diabetes mellitus: NIDDM or adult onset diabetes mellitus) or type 2 diabetes. Over 90 % of diabetics have type 2 diabetes and the remaining 10 % type 1. Other less prevalent types of diabetes mellitus include malnutrition-related diabetes mellitus (MRDM) and gestational diabetes mellitus (GDM).

Early signs of diabetes may include, excessive thirst and urination, tingling or numbness in the extremities, blurring of vision, muscle loss and occasionally excessive eating. The end result is that diabetes mellitus is a life-spoiling disease and one that shortens life expectancy if not properly managed. The causes and abnormal body functions leading to hyperglycemia, however, are markedly different among patients with diabetes mellitus, dictating different prevention strategies, diagnostic screening methods and treatments (Mayfield, 1998).

Diagnosis of Diabetes Mellitus

The diagnostic criterion for diabetes mellitus is a fasting plasma glucose (FPG) concentration of 7.0 mmol/L or 126 mg/dL and above (Table 1). For whole blood the proposed new level is 6.1 mmol/L or 110 mg/dL and above (WHO/ADA Expert Committee, 2003).
The diagnosis should not be based on a single glucose determination but requires confirmatory symptoms or blood/plasma determination. Ideally, both the 2-hour value in the 75g oral glucose tolerance test (OGTT) and the fasting value should be used (Alberti et al, 1999). If a diagnosis is made, the clinician must feel confident that the diagnosis is fully established since the consequences for the individual are considerable and lifelong.

Gestational diabetes mellitus (GDM) is diagnosed by a fasting plasma glucose level >126 mg/dl (7.0 mmol/L) or optimally an OGTT during pregnancy.

Table 1: Diagnosis of DM with a 100-g or 75-g glucose load

Treatment	Time	Plasma Gluscose Concentration	
		mg/dL	*mmol/L*
100-g Glucose Load	*Fasting*	95	7.0
	1-h	180	10.0
	2-h	155	8.6
	3-h	140	7.8
75-g Glucose Load	*Fasting*	95	7.0
	1-h	180	10.0
	2-h	155	8.6

Adapted from the American Diabetes Association, (2005)

Type 1 Diabetes Mellitus

Type 1 diabetes mellitus, formerly referred to as IDDM or juvenile onset diabetes mellitus, is characterized by destruction of the pancreatic beta cells arising from a cellular-mediated autoimmune process (Atkinson and Maclaren, 1994). This occurs when the immune system mistakenly manufactures antibodies that are directed against and cause damage to the pancreas, gradually leading to absolute insulin deficiency. Usually at least one or more of these autoantibodies are present in 85–90 % of individuals when fasting hyperglycemia is initially detected. It is believed that the tendency to develop these abnormal antibodies in type 1 diabetes is, in part, genetically inherited, though the details are not fully understood.

Exposure to certain viral infections such as mumps and Coxsackie viruses or other environmental toxins may serve to trigger abnormal antibody responses that cause damage to the pancreatic beta cells where insulin is synthesized. This subgroup is referred to as latent autoimmune diabetes in adults (LADA) and is a slow, progressive form of type 1 diabetes. In fact, LADA accounts for over 95% of those affected with type 1 diabetes mellitus and tend to occur in young, lean individuals; usually before 25 years of age, with an equal incidence in both sexes (Mayfield, 1998). However, older patients do show up with this form of diabetes on occasions. Individuals with this form of type 1 diabetes often become dependent on insulin for survival eventually and are at risk for ketoacidosis (Willis et al, 1996).

There are other classifications of type 1 diabetes mellitus referred to as the idiopathic form, which have no known etiology. Those affected have diminishing insulin secretion "insulinopenia" and are prone to ketoacidosis, but have no evidence of autoimmunity (McLarty et al, 1990). Although only a minority of patients with type 1diabetes fall into this category, the idiopathic form is more common among individuals of African and Asian origin (Mayfield, 1998; Alberti et al, 1999). In another form found mainly in the African diaspora, an absolute requirement for insulin replacement therapy in affected patients may be phasic, and patients rarely develop ketoacidosis (Ahrén and Corrigan, 1984). First described by Morrison, 1980, this form of diabetes is strongly inherited and lacks immunological evidence for ß-cell autoimmunity.

Noteworthy is the absolute requirement for insulin replacement therapy in affected patients intermittently. These patients show marked tolerability and asymptomatically accommodate very high blood sugar levels and are prone to kidney failure and early death

Type 2 Diabetes Mellitus

Type 2 diabetes mellitus formerly referred to as NIDDM or adult onset diabetes mellitus (AODM) is characterized by diabetics having relative, rather than absolute insulin deficiency. Type 2 diabetes mellitus is a heterogeneous syndrome of multiple gene "polygenic" origin and involves both defects in insulin secretion and insulin resistance (Defronzo et al, 1997). Even though insulin is produced, the body is either unable to regulate blood glucose levels or the amount of insulin produced is insufficient to normalize blood glucose levels. This form of diabetes frequently goes undiagnosed for many years as the hyperglycemia is often not severe enough to provoke noticeable symptoms of diabetes (Mooy et al, 1995; Harris, 1993). Nevertheless, such patients are at increased risk of developing cardiovascular complications (Mooy et al, 1995; Harris, 1993).

The risk of developing type 2 diabetes increases with age, obesity and lack of exercise (Zimmet, 1992) and has also been linked to familial genetics (de Courten et al, 1997; Knowler et al, 1993). Obesity itself causes some degree of insulin resistance and is one of the environmental factors in the development of type 2 diabetes (Ragoobirsingh et al, 2004). However, while it is said that type 2 diabetes mellitus occurs mostly in individuals over 30 years old and the incidence increases with age, there is an alarming increase in the prevalence of type 2 diabetes in children and adolescents (Soltesz, 2006). Type 2 diabetes mellitus occurs more frequently in women with prior GDM, individuals with hypertension or dyslipidemia, and persons of African descent and Hispanics.

Gestational Diabetes Mellitus

Gestational diabetes mellitus is characterized as carbohydrate intolerance resulting in hyperglycemia of variable severity with onset or first recognition during pregnancy (WHO, 1985; Alberti et al, 1999). The definition applies irrespective of whether insulin or only diet modification is used for treatment (American Diabetes Association, 2005). It does not exclude the possibility that unrecognized glucose intolerance may have antedated or begun concomitantly with the pregnancy. Women who become pregnant and who are known to have diabetes mellitus which antedates pregnancy are not classified as having GDM (WHO, 1999).

In healthy pregnant women, insulin is produced in large amounts, leading to increased rates of secretion. When this happens, women with an ineffective pancreas may not be able to manufacture the required amounts of insulin and therefore give rise to GDM (Stoffel et al, 1993; Coustan, 1995). In most women diagnosed with GDM, the associated abnormal glucose metabolism reverts to normal after the gestation period, but most are at an increased risk of subsequently developing type 2 diabetes mellitus (Benjamin et al, 1986; Saker et al, 1996).

Individuals at high risk for GDM include older women, those with previous history of glucose intolerance, women from certain high-risk ethnic groups such as African descent, Hispanics and Native Americans, and any pregnant woman with elevated fasting, or casual blood glucose levels (Alberti et al, 1999). Formal systematic testing for GDM is usually done between 24 and 28 weeks of the gestation period.

Other Specific Types

Other specific types currently include less common causes of diabetes mellitus, but are those in which the underlying defect or disease process can be identified in a relatively specific manner. They include, for example, fibrocalculous pancreatopathy, which is a disorder of the exocrine pancreas; a form of diabetes which was formerly classified as one type of malnutrition-related diabetes mellitus (WHO, 1999). Several other forms of diabetes are associated with monogenetic defects in ß-cell function. These forms of diabetes are frequently characterized by onset of hyperglycemia at an early age (Fajans and Bell, 2000). They are referred to as maturity-onset diabetes of the young (MODY) and are characterized by impaired insulin secretion with minimal or no defects in insulin action (WHO, 1999; American Diabetes Association, 2005).

Prevalence of Diabetes Mellitus

Diabetes mellitus is the most common chronic endocrine disorder; affecting an estimated 37.7 million adults aged 20—79 years in North America and the Caribbean region. It is expected that by 2030 the number of diabetes cases in the region will increase by 36 % or by over 13 million new cases (IDF, 2011). The accompanying shift in life-style to more sedentary activity with higher fat, lower fiber diets and resultant obesity, apparently underlies much of the increased prevalence of type 2 diabetes (Rewers and Hamman, 1995). The prevalence of diabetes for all age-groups worldwide was estimated at 8.8% in 2011 and expected to reach 9.9 % in 2030. This represents a projected rise in the number of adults with diabetes from the current 366 million to 552 million by 2030 (IDF, 2011). This increasing prevalence of diabetes is rapidly becoming a global lifestyle epidemic and as such adequate preventive and control methods must be enforced.

The National Health and Nutrition Examination Survey (NHANES) 1999-2000 report, indicated that a total of 8.3 % of persons aged >20 years had both diagnosed or undiagnosed diabetes and 19.2 % for persons aged >60 years (Mokdad et al, 2000). The study showed that men and women were equally affected by diabetes. Non-Hispanic blacks and Mexican Americans had a higher prevalence compared with non-Hispanic whites. Additionally, over 6 % of adults had impaired fasting glucose; representing 12.3 million people, increasing to 14.4 % for persons aged >60 years, with men affected more than women (Mokdad et al, 2000). Overall, an estimated 14.4 % of the U.S. population aged >20 years and 33.6 % of those aged >60 years had either diabetes or impaired fasting glucose (Center for Disease Control and Prevention, 2003).

As middle-income countries of the Caribbean undergo epidemiologic transition to chronic disease in ethnic minorities as in industrialized countries, diabetes mellitus has become a major public health concern (Wilks et al, 1999; Mbanya et al, 1999). Excessive diabetes complications exist among Afro-Americans and Afro-Caribbeans, who experience loss of vision, lower extremity amputation and end-stage renal disease at rates 1.5 to 4 fold higher than seen among comparable white groups (Kahn and Hiller, 1974; Most and Sinnock, 1983; Cowie et al, 1989; Harris, 1990).

In the year 2000, the number of people who suffered from diabetes in the Americas was estimated at 35 million, of which 19 million (54 %) lived in Latin America and the Caribbean (Figure 1). The projections indicate that by 2025 this number will increase to 64 million, of which 40 million (62 %) will live in Latin America and the Caribbean (King et al, 1998). This rising trend is observed in a number of Caribbean countries. Between 1971 and 2000 glucose intolerance in Cuba increased from 8.4 % to 24.8 % among the adult population (threefold increase in just under 30 years). In Jamaica, the prevalence of diabetes among persons 25–74 years old is estimated to be between 12 % and 16 % (Wilks et al, 1999; Cooper et al, 1997; Ragoobirsingh et al, 1995). In Latin America and the Caribbean, the highest prevalence rate was registered in Jamaica (17.9 %), and the lowest in Cuba with 11.8 %. In the majority of the countries, the prevalence of diabetes was higher in women than men.

However alarming these statistics may seem, recent studies have indicated that the prevalence of diabetes is still increasing in Caribbean countries. Hennis et al (2002) reported that the prevalence of diabetes in Barbados stood at 17 % of known diabetes cases; an increase of 3.5 % of the previously reported figure by Foster et al (1993). Diabetes prevalence (primarily type 2) varied with ethnic group, affecting 17.5 % of black, 12.5 % of mixed, and 6.0 % of white/other ethnic groups in Barbados (Hennis et al, 2002).

The increase in the prevalence of diabetes can be attributed to the rapid cultural and social changes, which are further amplified by the progressive migration of rural populations to cities and assimilation of habits that favor obesity. Another factor contributing to the high prevalence of diabetes mellitus is the increased consumption of complex carbohydrates with high glycemic indices (Bahado-Singh et al, 2011; 2006 and Riley & Bahado-Singh et al, 2008). This represents a shift from traditional cultures where the diet was comprised mainly of starchy low glycemic index (GI) carbohydrate foods (Jenkins et al, 1980b; Jenkins et al, 1986a; Ebbeling et al, 2005). It appears that the traditional use of low GI carbohydrate foods in the diet was particularly prevalent among cultures that are now experiencing high rates of diabetes, for example, the Pima

Indians and Caribbean nations, and where the change to high GI foods has been a more recent phenomenon (Thorburn et al, 1987; O'Dea, 1991; Boyce and Swimburn, 1993). Other factors, such as rising obesity; especially now in children and adolescents in the U.S.A. and the Caribbean, and reduced physical activity, play major roles in increasing diabetes risk.

Figure 1: Adjusted[1] prevalence rates of diabetes mellitus in adults in selected countries of the Americas (%)

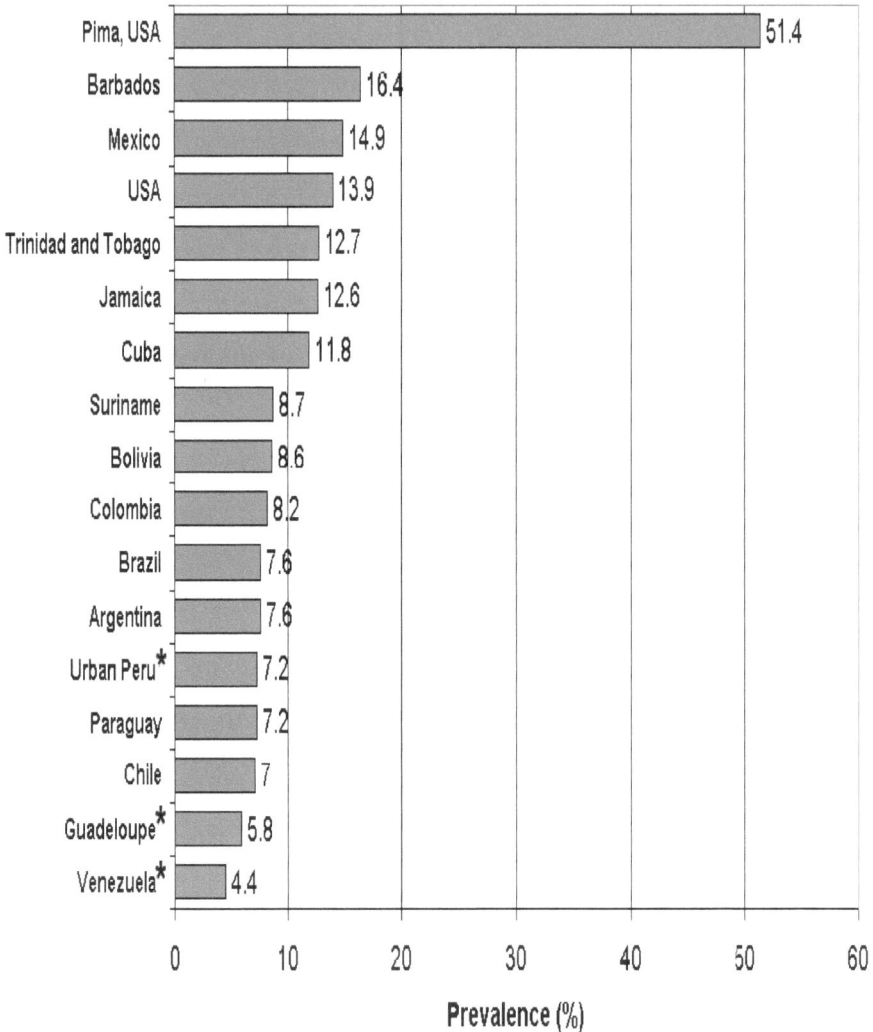

[1] Adjusted by direct method using the world population (Segi) as standard

* Crude rate

(Adapted from the Barceló, 2001)

Socio-Economic Impact of Diabetes Mellitus

Diabetes mellitus presents a high social and economic burden on individuals and the society. This burden is not only related to health care costs, but also indirectly, resulting in loss of productivity due to disability and premature mortality. Medical expenditures for persons with diabetes are 2-3 times higher than those not affected by the disease (Rubin et al, 1994).

The economic burden of diabetes mellitus is enormous and accounted for 11% of total global healthcare expenditures in 2011 (IDF 2011). This amounted to over $465 billion in expenditure in 2011, and is expected to exceed $595 billion by 2030. In 2011, the USA spent over $201 billion or 43% of global healthcare expenditure on diabetes and its complications. This is a marked increase in expenditure when compared to the 98 billion spent in 1997 (American Diabetes Association, 1998). In 1997, direct medical expenditures attributable to diabetes totaled $44.1 billion and comprised $7.7 billion for diabetes and acute glycemic care, $11.8 billion due to the excess prevalence of related chronic complications, and $24.6 billion due to the excess prevalence of general medical conditions (American Diabetes Association, 1998). The majority of attributable expenditures were for inpatient care (62 %), followed by outpatient services (25%) and nursing home care (13 %). Two-thirds of all medical costs for diabetes were borne by the elderly. Attributable indirect costs totaled $54.1 billion and comprised $17.0 billion resulting from premature mortality and $37.1 billion from disability (American Diabetes Association, 1998).

In 2002, the estimated medical costs associated with diabetes mellitus in the U.S. increased by over 25% from 1997. Direct medical and indirect expenditures attributable to diabetes in 2002 were estimated at US$132 billion (American Diabetes Association, 2003). Direct medical expenditures alone increased by over 50% from 1997, a total US$91.8 billion and comprised US$23.2 billion for diabetes care, US$24.6 billion for chronic complications attributable to diabetes, and US$44.1 billion for excess prevalence of general medical conditions. Attributable indirect expenditures resulting from lost workdays, restricted activity days, mortality, and permanent disability due to diabetes totaled US$39.8 billion (American Diabetes Association, 2003).

Studies done by the World Health Organization in 2003 revealed that the total cost attributed to diabetes mellitus for health care expenditures in the English speaking Caribbean countries exceeds US$1 billion. Jamaica alone accounts for almost a half of the reported figure totaling more than US$409 million (Barceló et al, 2003). A 2004 study revealed that diabetes cases in Jamaica have risen in excess of 300,000 in a population just fewer than 3 million. The 15 and over age group accounted for 17.9 % of the reported cases (Ragoobirsingh et al, 1995), and an additional 1.7 % diagnosed with impaired glucose tolerance (Ragoobirsingh et al, 2004). Alarmingly, diabetes mellitus is the second leading cause of death in Jamaica, accounting for 10 % of mortality (Statistical Institute of Jamaica, 1996). However, the impact of diabetes on mortality is under reported since the disease may contribute to mortality from other conditions such as cerebrovascular accidents and myocardial infarctions (Alleyne et al, 1989).

The health care expenditure for the Spanish speaking Caribbean countries in 2003 was almost twice that of the English speaking countries amounting to over US$2 billion (Barceló et al, 2003). The combined healthcare expenditure for the Caribbean exceeded $ 22 billion in 2011 indicating a 7 fold increase in the economic cost of the disease (IDF 2011). In Latin America and the Caribbean the annual number of deaths in 2000 caused by diabetes mellitus was estimated at 339,035. This represented a loss of 757,096 discounted years of productive life among persons younger than 65 years (>US$3 billion). Permanent disability caused a loss of 12,699,087 years and over US$50 billion, and temporary disability caused a loss of 136,701 years in the working population and over US$763 billion. The total annual cost associated with diabetes was estimated as US$65,216 million-direct cost US$10,721; indirect US$54,496 (Barceló et al, 2003). This is expected to further burden the healthcare systems which are already stretched by the AIDS/HIV pandemic in the Caribbean.

The vast financial burden of diabetes mellitus is the associated complications; blindness, kidney failure, amputations, and cardiovascular disease, which reduces the quality and length of life (Humphrey et al, 1994; Klein et al,

1995; Geiss et al, 1997). In the Caribbean and Latin America diabetes complications were responsible for more than 35 million medical visits annually (Barceló et al, 2003). As many as 1.8 million people were affected with heart disease, and a similar number affected by retinopathy. Nephropathy affected 0.8 million people with diabetes, neuropathy, 1.1 million and peripheral vascular disease 0.8 million. Overall, complications of diabetes were responsible for costs of more than US$2.4 billion. The highest cost was attributed to nephropathy US$1.8 billion; this was followed by retinopathy US$267 million and cardiovascular diseases amounted to more than US$240 million (Barceló et al, 2003). Diabetic nephropathy, progressing from the earliest stages of glomerular hyperfiltration and hypertrophy to micro-albuminuria (urinary albumin excretion, 30–300 mg/24 hr), clinical proteinuria (>300 mg albumin excretion/24 hours), and inexorably to end-stage renal failure, is the diabetes-specific complication that carries the most morbidity, mortality, and expense (Nathan, 2002).

As the global diabetes epidemic continues to unfold, experts have asked whether the war against it is being lost (King et al, 1998; Clark, 1998; Safran et al, 1999). Even though the socio-economic impact is catastrophic and overwhelming, it is never too late to implement adequate management strategies, geared towards sustaining life and equally reducing and preventing any further global financial burden of diabetes mellitus.

2 Management of Diabetes Mellitus

Overview

The prevention or reduction of diabetic complications in the diabetic population is the most imminent issue in the field of clinical diabetology. The burning question is how to solve or manage this rising dilemma. Glycemic control has proven to be the most effective means of preventing diabetic complications (Kikkawa et al, 2000). The importance of glycemic control has been confirmed by several large-scale controlled trials such as the DCCT (Diabetes Control and Complications Trial Research Group, 1993), the UKPDS (United Kingdom Prospective Diabetes Study Group, 1998) and Ohkubo et al (1995) study. These studies show that diabetics and individuals at high risk, who keep their blood glucose under tight control have reduced complications that results from this disease (Gilbertson et al, 2001). Studies have shown that one way of achieving glycemic control is through the intervention of medical and pharmacological innovations. These studies have shown that delaying the onset and slowing the progression of the disease are beneficial in mitigating associated clinical and cost repercussions (Harris, 1998b).

In the UKPDS, the preventive effects of various therapeutic agents (pharmaceutical drugs) on diabetic complications were compared; the findings indicated that glycemic control by any means is able to prevent diabetic complications. The development of the therapeutic forms of insulin (from pigs-porcine insulin and genetically engineered insulin-identical to human insulin) has gained tremendous popularity and efficacy in controlling hyperglycemia (Eventov-Friedman et al, 2005). For those affected with type 1 diabetes, daily insulin therapy (even continuous insulin infusion with external pumps) is essential to achieve near-normal glycemia (Renard,

2004; Owen, 2006). To a lesser extent, and only in extreme circumstances when diet and exercise does not work, insulin is used in the treatment of those with type 2 diabetes and GDM (Fox et al, 2006).

Pharmacological Management of Diabetes Mellitus

In making therapeutic choices in the management of type 2 diabetes, the major goal of protecting patients from the long-term complications of the disease must be considered. Because insulin resistance plays a fundamental role in the pathogenesis of type 2 diabetes and especially its adverse cardiovascular outcomes, interventions should initially be aimed towards improvement in tissue insulin sensitivity. This often involves the use of pharmacological therapy which targets specific tissues in the body (Figure 2). These therapeutic drugs can also improve many of the cardiovascular risk parameters of the metabolic syndrome.

Pharmaceutical therapies can include both intravenous and orally administered agents. Orally administered therapeutic drugs are often referred to as oral hypoglycemic agents or oral antihyperglycemic agents. Currently there are five classes of oral diabetes medications, all of which help in lowering blood glucose levels. The mechanism of action for the drugs may vary from stimulating insulin production to slowing down the absorption of carbohydrates in the intestines. The class of antidiabetic agents used will depend on several factors such as; the patients age, nature of diabetes (etiology), degree of control, among others. The different classes of diabetes medications can be used in combination or with insulin to achieve blood glucose control.

Classes and actions of medications:
- Thiazolidinediones: increase the body's sensitivity to insulin

- Biguanides: shuts off excess glucose production

- Sulfonylureas: stimulate the pancreas to make more insulin.

- Alpha-Glucosidase Inhibitors: slow absorption of carbohydrates in the intestine

- Meglitinides: stimulate the pancreas to make more insulin

- Incretins: stimulate pancreas to produce insulin (eg. GLP-1)

- DPP-4 inhibitors: stimulate pancreas to produce insulin by deactivating DPP

Figure 2: Pharmacological treatment of hyperglycemia according to site of action

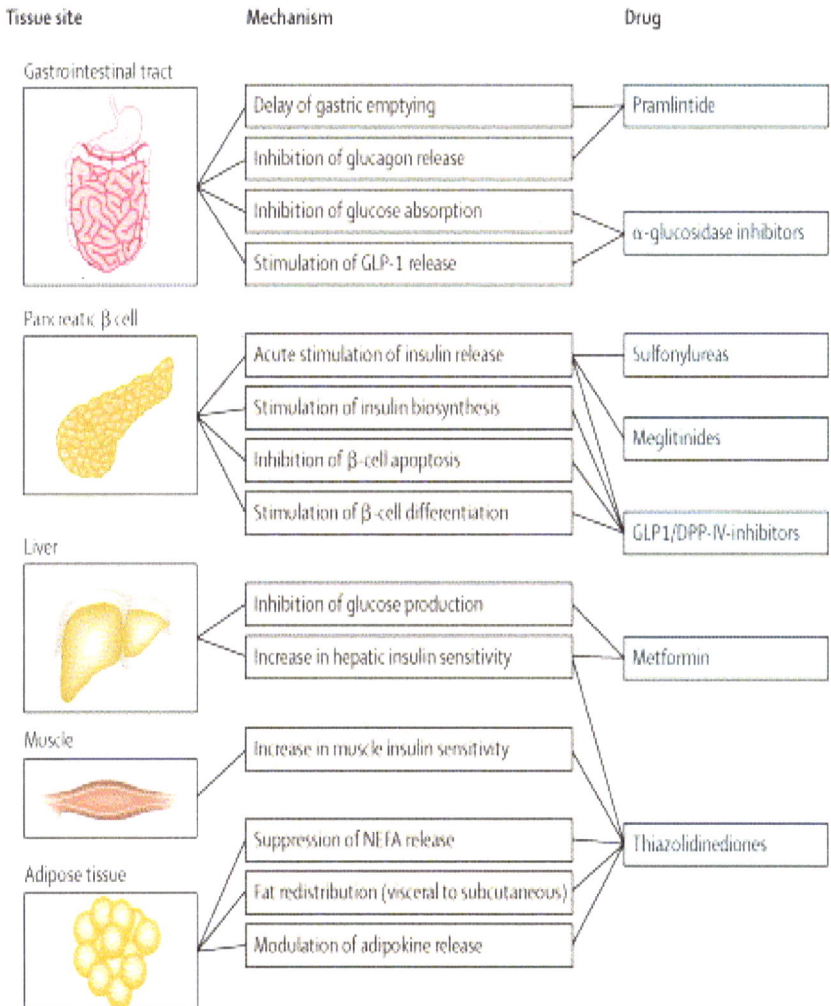

Tissue site	Mechanism	Drug
Gastrointestinal tract	Delay of gastric emptying	Pramlintide
	Inhibition of glucagon release	
	Inhibition of glucose absorption	α-glucosidase inhibitors
	Stimulation of GLP-1 release	
Pancreatic β cell	Acute stimulation of insulin release	Sulfonylureas
	Stimulation of insulin biosynthesis	Meglitinides
	Inhibition of β-cell apoptosis	
	Stimulation of β-cell differentiation	GLP1/DPP-IV-inhibitors
Liver	Inhibition of glucose production	
	Increase in hepatic insulin sensitivity	Metformin
Muscle	Increase in muscle insulin sensitivity	
Adipose tissue	Suppression of NEFA release	Thiazolidinediones
	Fat redistribution (visceral to subcutaneous)	
	Modulation of adipokine release	

Adapted from Stumvoll et al, 2005

Thiazolidinediones (glitazones)

Insulin sensitivity can be enhanced by pharmacological drugs; primarily those of the thiazolidinedione class (also known as glitazones). This class of drugs not only reduces glycemia, but enhances vascular function and ameliorates the dyslipidaemia and inflammatory milieu of type 2 diabetes. Thiazolidinediones primarily activate PPAR (peroxisome proliferator-activated receptors) receptors in adipose tissue and alter adipose metabolism and distribution. They also reduce circulating concentrations of pro-inflammatory cytokines that promote insulin resistance and at the same time increase concentrations of adiponectin, which has insulin-sensitizing and anti-inflammatory properties. The multiple effects of thiazolidinediones on adipose tissue metabolism and cross-talk of these signals with liver and skeletal muscle, as well as pancreatic beta-cells and the vascular endothelium, might account for the enhancement of insulin action and improvement in insulin secretion with these agents, as well as several beneficial effects on vascular function (Meriden, 2004).

The thiazolidinediones, unlike the biguanides such as metformin, can be used in patients with reduced renal function without significant gastrointestinal side-effects. A major adverse effect associated with clinical use of the thiazolidinediones is weight gain, which seems to be coupled to the effects of the drugs on adipose cell differentiation and triglyceride storage. Fluid retention is also linked to the activity of the thiazolidinediones resulting in peripheral oedema and a mild haemodilution in some patients. Fortunately, congestive heart failure is quite rare with use of thiazolidinediones, but remains a serious concern that requires caution in selection of patients to receive these agents (Nesto et al, 2003). The ability of thiazolidinediones to ameliorate risk of atherosclerotic events is being assessed in several large outcomes studies. The most commonly prescribed thiazolidinediones (glitazones) includes; rosiglitazone (Avandia), and Pioglitazone (Actos).

Biguanides

Biguanides such as Metformin are highly effective anti-hyperglycemic drugs that work independently of the pancreas, sparing insulin (Lord et al, 2006). Metformin reduces the overproduction of glucose by the liver. It helps in lowering the blood sugar, especially after eating, with no risk of hypoglycemia when used alone. It decreases hepatic glucose output and has been shown to have a beneficial effect on cardiovascular outcomes (Bailey and Turner, 1996; Cusiet et al, 1996; Mamputu et al, 2003). Owing to the fact that metformin shuts off the liver's production of excess glucose, it reduces the amount of injected insulin required to control the blood sugar levels in both Type 1 and Type 2 diabetes. Type 2 diabetics on insulin are usually advised to lower their insulin doses prior to starting metformin. Metformin has less robust effects on insulin resistance, inflammatory markers, and vascular function compared with the thiazolidinediones, but its benefit in abrogating some of the weight gain commonly observed with insulin-sensitizers and insulin secretion enhancers adds important value to this drug (Topcu et al, 2006).

Side effects from metformin may include changes in taste, loss of appetite, nausea or vomiting, abdominal bloating or gas, diarrhea, or skin rash. Taking the medication with food and starting out with a low dose may help to reduce side effects. The dosage can be gradually increased as side effects diminish.

Sulfonylureas

As inadequate beta-cell insulin secretion is fundamental to the development of hyperglycemia in diabetes, insulin secretion enhancers also play an important role in control of blood glucose (Mori et al, 2006). Sulfonylureas act by closing pancreatic cell potassium channels leading to enhanced insulin secretion (Huang et al, 2006). The mode of action of sulfonylureas implies that they also act on low concentrations of plasma glucose, which explains the potential of hypoglycemia (occasionally severe). Sulfonylurea derivatives normally result in moderate decreases in plasma glucose concentrations in most patients with type 2 diabetes and reduction of glycated hemoglobin (Hb A1c) concentrations (Stumvoll et al, 2005). Some sulfonylureas such as tolbutamide, gliclazide, and glipizide have relatively short durations of action (3 hours), while others like glimepiride and glibenclamide (glyburide) are long acting (24 hr), adding to the risk of hypoglycemia (Rendell, 2004).

The results of the UK Prospective Diabetes Study (1998) showed clear risk reduction in microvascular complications and

16 % reduction in macrovascular diseases when sulfonylurea derivatives are used. Combined management with both sulfonylurea derivatives and antihypertensives improves the risk reduction even more (Hannan et al, 2006; Coca et al, 2006). Some of the most widely used branded sulfonylureas used in diabetes management include; Tolinase, Diabinese, Pres Tab, Glycotrol, Amaryl (Glimepiride) and Diabeta.

Alpha-Glucosidase Inhibitors

Alpha-glucosidase inhibitors also referred to as starch blockers aid in the control of plasma glucose concentrations by slowing down the digestion of complex carbohydrates and as such, significantly reduces postprandial glucose spikes and fasting blood glucose levels.

The mechanism of action of Alpha-glucosidase inhibitors is different from other oral hypoglycemic drugs as they act by inhibiting enzymes in the intestine that are responsible for carbohydrate digestion. They slow down the activity of the enzymes resulting in slower glucose uptake in the blood with a resulting lower blood glucose concentration.

The two major Alpha-Glucosidase inhibitors used are Precose (Acarbose) and Glyset (Miglitol). These drugs are taken with every meal.

Meglitinides

Meglitinides acts by increasing insulin levels via stimulation of pancreatic beta cells. The mechanism of action is believed to be different from that of sulfonylureas. They enhance insulin release from the pancreas over a short period of time and only act when the blood glucose levels are high. Meglitinides have a shorter action than sulfonylureas, and are associated with lower risk of hypoglycemia. Additionally, they can also be used in patients with decreased renal function (Rendell, 2004).

The two most commonly used Meglitinides are Prandin (Repaglinide) and Starlix (nateglinide) and are usually taken 10 to 15 minutes before meals. Like sulfonylureas, they do not work in Type 1 diabetes and require beta cells capable of producing insulin. Both drugs bind to the same site of sulphonylurea receptor 1 as do the sulfonylurea derivatives, and repaglinide, which binds to a nearby site of the receptor (Mandic and Gabelica, 2006), both leading to insulin release. These agents cannot further stimulate insulin release in patients on maximal doses of sulfonylurea derivatives.

In patients who retain residual insulin production, one of these medications can be combined with basal insulin such as NPH (Neutral Protamine Hagedorn), Levemir, or Lantus to provide better control. The injected insulin provides basal coverage to keep the fasting blood sugar at a good level, while one of the rapid insulin releasers can enhance internal insulin release to control the blood sugar after meals.

Incretins and DPP-4 Inhibitors

Incretins are gastrointestinal hormones secreted from enteroendocrine cells into the blood within minutes after eating. Their main role is to regulate the amount of insulin secreted by the pancreas. The two main incretins of interest are glucose-dependent insulinotropic peptide (GIP) and glucagon-like peptide-1 (GLP-1). GLP-1 acts to stimulate insulin release from the pancreatic β-cells, suppress glucagon release from the pancreatic β-cells, slow gastric emptying, and increase satiety. However, both hormones are believed to share similar roles in the pancreas but have distinct actions outside of the pancreas (Kim and Egan, 2008).

A lack of secretion of incretins or increases in their clearance is not a pathogenic factor in diabetes. However, GIP no longer modulates glucose-dependent insulin secretion in type 2 diabetics, and can be detrimental to β-cell function, especially after eating. GLP-1, on the other hand, is still insulinotropic in type 2 diabetics. This has led to the development of several pharmaceutical agents that can activate the GLP-1 receptor in a bid to improving insulin secretion. As such two major classes of drugs based on incretin action have been developed and are currently being used for lowering blood glucose levels in type 2 diabetics. These include Dipeptidyl peptidase 4 resistant analogues such as exenatide (potent long-acting agonist of the GLP-1 receptor) and GLP-1 enhancer/DPP 4 inhibitors such as sitagliptin.

Exenatide is injected subcutaneously twice daily and results in lower blood glucose and higher insulin levels. There is heavy glucose-dependency to its secretory capacity, and as such is unlikely to induce hypoglycemic episodes. DPP4 inhibitors on the other hand are orally administered and result in increases in endogenous active incretin levels in the blood, thus leading to prolonged incretin action (Kim and Egan, 2008).

Exogenous insulin

Insulin is among the oldest and the most effective treatment in controlling blood glucose levels. Additionally, it has been the most effective treatment in diabetes owing to its ability to control any degree of hyperglycemia in type 1 or type 2 diabetics. Even though it was initially prepared by isolation from animal pancreatic tissue, insulin is now predominantly prepared through recombinant DNA techniques. As such, the primary source of exogenous insulin such as humulin from Eli Lilly and analogues such as Lispro (Elli Lilly), aspart (Novo Nordisk) and glulisine (Sanofi Aventis) are synthesized. In 2002 the International Diabetes Federation reported that over 70% of the insulin sold in the world was recombinant or biosynthetic 'human' insulin (IDF 2004). Insulin has been classified into four categories based on their mode of action, namely:

- **Rapid-acting:** begins to work after 15 minutes, peaks in 30—90 minutes, and last for 3—4 hours.

- **Short-acting:** begins to work in 30—60 minutes, peaks in 2—3 hours, and last for 3—6 hours.

- **Intermediate-acting:** begins to work in 90 minutes —6 hours, peaks in 4—14 hours, and last for up to 24 hours.

- **Long-acting:** begins to work in 6—14 hours and remains effective for 24—36 hours.

Insulin may be administered transdermally (via micro-jets), subcutaneously (via syringe), via inhalation or insulin pump. Clinical trials are currently ongoing to assess the efficacy of oral and transnasal insulin delivery systems.

Owing to the loss of ß-cell function in type 1 diabetics

and absolute insulin deficiency the basis of therapy is insulin treatment. However, because type 1 diabetes does not affect insulin sensitivity, patients usually require only small doses of insulin to maintain glucose control. Type 2 diabetes, on the other hand, is characterized by insulin resistance followed by relative insulin deficiency. As such patients with type 2 diabetes tend to require higher doses of insulin and an incremental increase in doses as the disease progresses.

Experimental approaches used in the Management of Diabetes Mellitus

As specific drug targets are identified through improved understanding of the molecular pathogenesis of diabetes, novel therapeutics will become available in the future. For example, PTP1B is a negative regulator of insulin signalling, and inhibition of its activity with specific pharmaceutical agents, or reduction of its protein concentrations with novel antisense oligonucoleotides, has been shown to enhance insulin action in pre-clinical models (Liu, 2004).

Controlling excessive secretion of interleukin 6 or blocking their action mediated by serine/threonine kinases would be expected to enhance insulin sensitivity in patients with visceral adiposity (Perregaux et al, 2001). Conversely, increasing adiponectin secretion or administration of an adiponectin receptor agonist would probably enhance glucose metabolism in skeletal muscle and liver and also confer beneficial effects in the endothelium. Recent evidence for amelioration of insulin resistance by salicylates by favorable interference with the inflammatory kinase cascade in insulin signalling might lead to entirely novel therapeutic approaches (Shoelson et al, 2003).

Nutrition in the management of Diabetes Mellitus

In spite of drug therapy, dietetic management is regarded as the backbone of the regulation and management of diabetes mellitus, particularly of type 2 diabetes, where the primary derangement is of carbohydrate metabolism (ADA, 2002). The recommendation to exercise and eat more fiber and less saturated and trans-fat is excellent advice (Wolever, 1990b) –

as far as it goes.

Studies have shown that the consumption of fiber reduces the rate of nutrient influx from the small intestine (Jenkins et al, 2002), which in turn reduces the glycemic response in diabetics. Reducing the consumption of saturated and trans-fat reduces the risk of developing cardiovascular diseases (Mozaffarian et al, 2004; Schulze and Hu, 2005). The Netherlands Health Council recommends a daily dietary intake of ‹10% saturated fatty acids and ‹1% trans-fatty acids of the total energy intake (Woodside and Kromhout, 2005). This has prompted the Food and Drug Administration (FDA) to issue new guidelines, as of the beginning of 2006, that trans-fat must be listed on food labels in the U.S. (Mozaffarian et al, 2006). In contrast, recent studies (Schulze and Hu, 2005; Mozaffarian et al, 2006) have shown increasing evidence that the quality of fat plays a more important role than does the quantity, and thus, public health strategies should emphasize replacing saturated and trans-fats; from the industrial food supply, with unsaturated fats.

References

Ahrén, B. and Corrigan, C.B. 1984. 'Intermittent need for insulin in a subgroup of diabetic patients in Tanzania'. Diabetic Medicine no.2: 262-64.

Alberti, K. Aschner, P. et. al. 1999. 'Definition, Diagnosis and Classification of Diabetes Mellitus and Its Complications, Part 1: Diagnosis and Classification of Diabetes Mellitus'. World Health Organization Technical Report Series, no. 99: 1-59.

American Diabetes Association. 2005. 'Diagnosis and Classification of Diabetes Mellitus'. Diabetes Care, no.28: S37-S42.

American Diabetes Association. 2003. 'Economic Costs of Diabetes in the U.S. in 2002'. Diabetes Care, no. 26: 917-932.

American Diabetes Association.1998. 'Economic consequences of Diabetes Mellitus in the U.S. in 1997'. Diabetes Care, no. 21: 296-309.

American Diabetes Association.1991. 'Nutritional recommendations and principles for individuals with diabetes mellitus. Diabetes Care, no.14 (2): 20-27.

Atkinson, M.A and Maclaren, N.K. 1994. 'The pathogenesis of insulin dependent diabetes'. New England Journal of Medicine, no.331: 1428-1436.

Bailey, C.J. and Turner, R.C. 1996 'Metformin'. New England Journal of Medicine, no. 334: 574-579.

Barceló, A. 2001. 'PAHO's Non-Communicable Diseases Program, Division of Disease Prevention and Control (HCP/HCN). Diabetes in the Americas'. Epidemiological bulletin Pan America Health Organization, no. 22 (2): 1-3.

Barceló, A. 2000. 'Diabetes and hypertension in the Americas'. West Indian Medical Journal. no.49 (4): 262-265.

Barceló, A., Aedo, C., Rajpathak, S. and Robles, S. 2003. 'The cost of diabetes in Latin American and the Caribbean'. Bulletin of the World Health Organization, no.81 (1): 19-27.

Benjamin, F., Wilson, S.J. et al. 1986. 'Effect of advancing pregnancy on the glucose tolerance test and on the 50-gram oral glucose screening test for gestational diabetes'. American Journal of Obstetrics and Gynecology, no.68: 362-365.

Boyce, V.L. and Swimburn, B.A. 1993 'The traditional Pima Indian diet. Composition and adaptation for use in a dietary intervention study'. Diabetes Care, no.16: 369-371.

Bahado-Singh, P.S., Cliff K. Riley. et al. 2011. 'Relationship between processing method and the glycemic indices of ten sweet potato (Ipomoea batatas) cultivars commonly consumed in Jamaica'. Journal of Nutrition & Metabolism, no. 10.1155/2011/584832

Bahado-Singh, P.S., Wheatley, A.O. et al. 2006. 'Food processing methods influence the glycemic indices of some commonly eaten West Indies carbohydrate-rich foods'.

British Journal of Nutrition, no.96 (3): 476-448.

Center for Disease Control and Prevention. 2003. 'Prevalence of Diabetes and Impaired Fasting Glucose in Adults - United States, 1999-2000', no.52 (35): 833-837.

Clark, C.M. 1998. 'How should we respond to the worldwide diabetes epidemic'? Diabetes Care, no. 21: 475–476.

Coca, A., Dalfo, A., Esmaties, E. et al.2006. 'Treatment and control of cardiovascular risk in primary care in Spain. The PREVENCAT study'. Journal of Clinical Medicine, no. 126(6): 201-205.

Cooper, R.S., Rotimi, C.N. et al. 1997. 'Prevalence of NIDDM among populations of the African diaspora'. Diabetes Care, no. 20(3): 343-348.

Coustan, D.R. 1995. 'Gestational diabetes'. Diabetes in America. 2nd Edition, no. 95-1468.

Cowie, C.C., Port, F.K., et al.1989. 'Disparities in incidence of diabetic end-stage renal disease according to race and type of diabetes'. New England Journal of Medicine, no. 321:1074–1079.

Cusiet, K., Consoli, A., and DeFronzo, R.A. 1996. 'Metabolic effects of metformin on glucose and lactate metabolism in non insulin-dependent diabetes mellitus'. Journal of Clinical Endocrinology and Metabolism, no 81: 4059-4067.

Deacon, C.F. 2004. 'Therapeutic strategies based on glucagon-like peptide 1'. Diabetes journals, no. 53: 2181–2189.

De Courten, M., Zimmet, P., Hodge, A., et al. 1997. 'Hyperleptinaemia: The missing link in the metabolic syndrome?' Diabetic Medicine, no. 14 (3): 200-208.

De Fronzo, R.A., Bonadonna, R.C., and Ferrannini, E. 1997. 'Pathogenesis of NIDDM'. International Textbook of Diabetes Mellitus. 2nd edition. Alberti KGMM, Zimmet, P. 635-712. Chichester: Wiley.

Diabetes Control and Complications Trial Research Group. 1993. 'The effect of intensive treatment of diabetes on the development and progression of long-term complications in insulin dependent diabetes mellitus'. New England Journal of Medicine, no 329: 977-986.

Ebbeling, C.B., Leidig, M.M. et al. 2005. 'Effects of ad libitum low-glycemic load diet on cardiovascular disease risk factors in obese young adults'. American Journal of Clinical Nutrition, no. 81(5): 976-982.

Eventov-Friedman, S., Katchman, H. et al. 2005. 'Embryonic pig liver, pancreas and lung as a source for transplantation: Optimal organogenesis without teratoma depends on distinct time windows'. Proceedings of the National Academy of Sciences, no. 102(8): 2928–2933.

Fajans, S.S. and Bell, G. 2000. 'Maturity onset diabetes of the young: a model for genetic studies of diabetes mellitus'. A fundamental and clinical text. 2nd edition. Le Roith D., Taylor S. I. And Olefsky, J.M. Eds. 691-705. Philadelphia.

Foster, C., Rotimi, C. Et al.1993. 'Hypertension, diabetes, and obesity in Barbados: findings from a recent population-based survey'. Ethnicity and Disease, no.3: 404-12.

Fox, K.M., Gerber-Pharmd, R.A. et al. 2006. 'Prevalence of inadequate glycemic control among patients with type 2 diabetes in the United Kingdom general practice research database: A series of retrospective analyses of data from 1998 through 2002'. Clinical Therapeutics, no.28 (3): 388-395.

Geiss, L.S., Engelgau, M., Frazier, E. and Tierney, E. 1997. 'Diabetes Surveillance. Atlanta, GA, Centers for Disease Control and Prevention'. U.S. Dept. of Health and Human Services, no. 84-109.

Gilbertson, H.R., Jennie, C. Et al. 2001. 'The effect of flexible low glycemic index dietary advice versus measured carbohydrate exchange diets on glycemic control in children with type 1 diabetes'. Diabetes Care, no. 24: 1137-1143.

Hannan, J.M., Marenah, L. Et al. 2006. 'Ocimum sanctum leaf extracts stimulate insulin secretion from perfused pancreas, isolated islets and clonal pancreatic beta-cells'. Journal of Endocrinology, no. 189(1): 127-130.

Harris, M. I. 1993. 'Undiagnosed NIDDM; clinical and public health issues'. Diabetes Care, no. 16: 642-652.

Harris, M.I. 1990. 'Non-insulin-dependent diabetes mellitus in black and white Americans'. Diabetes Metabolism Review, no. 6: 71–90.

Humphrey, L.L., Palumbo, P.J.et al. 1994. 'The contribution of non-insulin-dependent diabetes to lower-extremity amputation in the community'. Archives of Internal Medicine, no. 154: 885–892.

International Diabetes Federation.2004. Diabetes Atlas: 2nd edition. Brussels.

International Diabetes Federation.2011. Diabetes Atlas: 5th edition. Brussels.

Jenkins, D.J.A, Kendall, C.W.C. et al. 2002. 'Glycemic index: Overview of implications in health and disease'. American Journal of Clinical Nutrition, no.76: Suppl., 237-266.

Jenkins, D.J., Wolever, T.M. et al.1986. 'Low glycemic response to traditionally processed wheat and rye products: bulgur and pumpernickel bread'. American Journal of Clinical Nutrition, no. 43: 516-520.

Jenkins, D.J., Wolever, T.M.et al. 1980. 'Exceptionally low blood glucose response to dried beans: comparison with other carbohydrate foods'. British Medical Journal, no. 281: 578-580.

Kahn, H.A. and Hiller, R. 1974. 'Blindness caused by diabetic retinopathy'. American Journal of Ophthalmology, no. 78: 58-67.

Kendall, D.M., Kim, D. and Maggs, D. 2006. 'Incretin Mimetics and Dipeptidyl Peptidase-IV Inhibitors: A review of emerging therapies for Type 2 Diabetes'. Diabetes Technology and Therapeutics, no.8 (3):385-396.

Kikkawa, R. 2000. Chronic complications in diabetes mellitus. British Journal of Nutrition, no. 84: S183-S185.

Kim, W. and Egan, J. 2008. 'The Role of Incretins in Glucose Homeostasis and Diabetes Treatment'. Pharmacological Reviews 60, no. 4: 470-512.

King, H., Aubert, R.E. and Herman, W.H. 1998. 'Global Burden of Diabetes'. Diabetes Care, no 21:1414-1431.

King, H. and Rewers, M. 1993. 'WHO Ad Hoc Diabetes Reporting Group. Global estimates for prevalence of diabetes mellitus and impaired glucose tolerance in adults'. Diabetes Care, no. 16:157–177.

Klein, R. and Klein, B.E.K. 1995. 'Vision disorders in diabetes'. Diabetes in America. 2nd edition. Harris, M.I., Cowie, C.C. et al, 95-1468. Washington DC. Government Printing Office.

Knowler, W.C., Saad, M.F. 1993. Determinants of Diabetes Mellitus in the Pima Indians. Diabetes Care 16: 216-227.

Liu, G. 2004. 'Technology evaluation: ISIS-113715, Isis'. Current Opinion in Molecular Therapeutics, no. 6: 331-336.

Mamputu, J.C., Wiernsperger, N.F. and Renier, G. 2003. 'Antiatherogenic properties of metformin: the experimental evidence'. Diabetes and Metabolism, no. 29: 71-76.

Mandic, Z. and Gabelica, V. 2006. 'Ionization, lipophilicity and solubility properties of repaglinide'. Journal of Pharmaceutical and Biomedical Analysis, no. 41(3): 866-871.

Mayfield, J. 1998. 'Diagnosis and Classification of Diabetes Mellitus: New Criteria'. American Family Physician journals, no. 58: 10-15.

Mbanya, J.C.N., Cruickshank, J.K., Forrester, T., et al. 1999. 'Standardised comparison of glucose intolerance in West African-origin populations or rural and urban Cameroon, Jamaica and Caribbean migrants to Britain'. Diabetes Care, no. 22: 434 - 440.

McLarty, D.G., Athaide, I. Et al. 1990. 'Islet cell antibodies are not specifically associated with insulin-dependent diabetes in rural Tanzanian Africans'. Diabetes Research and Clinical Practice, no. 9: 219 - 224.

Meriden, T. 2004. 'Progress with thiazolidinediones in the management of type 2 diabetes mellitus', Clinical Therapeutics, no. 26: 177-190.

Mokdad, A.H., Ford, E.S. et al. 2000. 'Diabetes Trends in the U.S.: 1990–1998', Diabetes Care, no. 23:1278 – 1283.

Mooy, J. M., Grootenhuis, P.A. et al.1995. 'Prevalence and determinants of glucose intolerance in a Dutch population. The Hoorn Study'. Diabetes Care, no. 18: 1270-1273.

Mori, Y., Itoh, Y., Obata, T. and Tajima, N. 2006. 'Effects of pioglitazone vs glibenclamide on postprandial increases in glucose and triglyceride levels and on oxidative stress in Japanese patients with type 2 diabetes'. Endocrine, no. 9(1):143 -148.

Most, R.S. and Sinnock, P. 1983. 'The epidemiology of lower extremity amputations in diabetic individuals'. Diabetes Care, no. 6: 87–91.

Mozaffarian, D., Pischon, T. 2004. 'Dietary intake of trans fatty acids and systemic inflammation in women'. American Journal of Clinical Nutrition ,no.79 (4): 606-612.

Nathan, D. M. 2002. 'The Impact of Clinical Trials on the Treatment of Diabetes Mellitus'. Journal of Clinical Endocrinology and Metabolism, no. 87(5): 1929-1937.

Nesto, R.W., Bell, D. and Bonow, R.O. 2003. 'Thiazolidinedione use, fluid retention, and congestive heart failure: a consensus statement from the American Heart Association and American Diabetes Association'. Circulation, no. 108: 2941-2948.

O'Dea, K. 1991. 'Westernisation, insulin resistance and diabetes in Australian aborigines'. Medical Journal of Australia, no. 155: 258-264.

Ohkubo, Y., Kishikawa, H. et al. 1995. 'Intensive insulin therapy prevents the progression of diabetic mircovascular complications in Japanese patients with non-insulin dependent diabetes mellitus: a randomized prospective 6-year study'. Diabetes Research and Clinical Practice, no. 28: 103-117.

Owen, S.K. 2006. 'Amylin replacement therapy in patients with insulin-requiring type 2 diabetes'. Diabetes Education, no. 32 (3): 105S-110S.

Perregaux, D.G., McNiff, P. et.al. 2001. 'Identification and characterization of a novel class of interleukin-1 post-translational processing inhibitors'. Journal of Pharmacology and Experimental Therapeutics, no. 299(1): 187 - 197.

Ragoobirsingh, D., Lewis-Fuller, F. and Morrison, E.Y. 1995. 'The Jamaican Diabetes Survey. A protocol for the Caribbean'. Diabetes Care, no. 18: 1277-1279.

Ragoobirsingh, D., Morrison, E.Y. et al. 2004. Obesity on the Caribbean: the Jamaican experience'. Diabetes, Obesity and Metabolism, no. 6: 23-27.

Renard, R. 2004. Implantable insulin delivery pumps. Journal of Minimally Invasive Therapy and Allied Technologies, no. 13(5):328-335.

Rendell, M. 2004. 'The role of sulfonylureas in the management of type 2 diabetes mellitus'. Drugs, no. 64: 1339-1358.

Rewers, M. and Hamman, R. 1995. 'Risk factors for non-insulin dependent diabetes'. Diabetes in America, 2nd Edition, no. 95: 79–230.

Riley, C.K., Bahado-Singh, P.S. et al. 2008. 'Relationship between the physicochemical properties of starches and the glycemic index of some Jamaican yams (Dioscorea spp.)'. Molecular Nutrition and Food Research, no. 52: 1372-1376.

Saker, P.J., Hattersley, A.T. and Barrow, B. 1996. 'High prevalence of a missense mutation of the glucokinase gene in gestational diabtes patients due to a founder-effect in a local population'. Diabetologia, no. 37: 104-110.

Schulze, M.B. and Hu, F.B. 2005. 'Primary prevention of diabetes: what can be done and how much can be prevented?' Annual Review of Public Health, no. 26: 445-467.

Shoelson, S.E., Lee, J. and Yuan, M. 2003. 'Inflammation and the IKK beta/I kappa B/NF-kappa B axis in obesity- and diet-induced insulin resistance'. International Journal of Obesity and Related Metabolic Disorders, no.27:S49-S52.

Soltesz G. 2006. 'Type 2 diabetes in children: An emerging clinical problem'. Diabetes Research and Clinical Practice, no. 74: S9-S11.

Statistical Institute of Jamaica .1996. 'Population census'. Statistical Institute of Jamaica, no. 1:15-61.

Stoffel, M., Bell, K.L. et.al.1993. 'Identification of glucokinase mutations in subjects with gestational diabetes mellitus'. Diabetes, no. 42: 937-940.

Stumvoll, M., Goldstein, B.J. and van Haeften, T.W. 2005. 'Type 2 diabetes: principles of pathogenesis and therapy'. Lancet, no. 365: 1333-1346.

The International Expert Committee. 2003. 'The Diagnosis and Classification of Diabetes Mellitus: Follow-up report on the diagnosis of diabetes mellitus'. Diabetes Care, no.26: 3160–3167.

Thorburn, A.W., Brand, J.C. and Truswell, A.S. 1987. 'Slowly digested and absorbed carbohydrate in traditional bushfoods: a protective factor against diabetes'? American Journal of Clinical Nutrition, no.45: 98–106.

UK Prospective Diabetes Study Group. 1998. 'Tight blood pressure control and risk of macrovascular and mircovascular complications in type 2 diabetes'. British Medical Journal, no. 317: 705-713.

Wild, S., Roglic, G., Sicree, R. and King, H. 2004. 'Global prevalence of diabetes: Estimates for the year 2000 and projections for 2030'. Diabetes Care, no. 27: 1047-1053.

Wilks, R.J, Rotimi C.N., Bennett, F., et al. 1999. 'Diabetes in the Caribbean: Results of a population survey from Spanish Town, Jamaica'. Diabetic Medicine, no. 16(10): 875-883.

Willis, J.A., Scott, R.S., Brown, L.J., et al. 1996. 'Islet cell antibodies and antibodies against glutamic acid decarboxylase in newly diagnosed adult-onset diabetes mellitus'. Diabetes Research and Clinical Practice, no. 33: 89-97.

Wolever, T. M. S. 1990b. 'Relationship between dietary fiber content and composition in foods and the glycemic index'. American Journal of Clinical Nutrition, no. 51: 72-75.

Woodside, J.V. and Kromhout, D. 2005. 'Fatty acids and CHD'. Proceedings of the Nutrition Society, no. 64(4): 554-564.

World Health Organization Study Group.1999. 'Definition, Diagnosis and Classification of Diabetes Mellitus and Its Complications, Part 1: Diagnosis and Classification of Diabetes Mellitus'. World Health Organization Technical Report Series, no. 99: 1-59.

World Health Organization Study Group.1985. 'Diabetes Mellitus: Report of a WHO Study Group'. World Health Organization Technical Report Series, no. 727:1-113.

Zimmet, P., Alberti, K.G. and Shaw, J. 2001. 'Global and societal implications of the diabetes epidemic'. Nature, no. 414: 782–787.

Zimmet, P.Z. 1992. 'Challenges in diabetes epidemiology (from West to rest)'. Diabetes Care, no.15(2): 232-252.

Zimmet, P., King, H. and Taylor, R. 1984. 'The high prevalence of diabetes mellitus, impaired glucose tolerance and diabetic retinopathy in Nauru'. Diabetes Research, no. 1: 13–18.

3

Plants used in
Diabetes Management
- Scientifically Validated

Overview of Scientific Studies on Caribbean Plants

Investigations into the medicinal properties of Jamaican and other Caribbean plants have been ongoing for several decades. The properties and efficacy of these natural remedies have also been a point of controversy among naturalist and western medicine practitioners because of the conservation concerns on one hand and questions about efficacy and toxicity on the other hand. There is also a social concern about the lack of robust scientific studies to support or dismiss such claims owing to the fact that little is known or has been translated to the general public and scientific community outlining the scientific validity of such claims. As a result of this, herbal therapies resulting from natural plant resources are not widely incorporated into modern day therapeutic management of a non communicable disease such as diabetes mellitus.

Despite these issues, the use of herbal medicines for the treatment of diabetes mellitus has gained medical and scientific importance throughout the world. The World Health Organization recommends and encourages the use of traditional therapies especially in countries where access to the conventional treatment of diabetes is not adequate (WHO, 1980). Studies have indicated that there is an increased demand for natural remedies with antidiabetic activity not only because of socio-economic issues but also due to the side effects associated with the use of insulin and oral hypoglycemic agents. The literature shows that over 400 plant species possess hypoglycemic activity (Oliver, 1986). However, despite the fact that these plants have a great reputation in the indigenous systems of medicine for their antidiabetic activities,

31

many remain to be scientifically evaluated for their bioactive chemical constituents and toxicity.

As early as 1955, Jones embarked on preliminary clinical trials to evaluate efficacy of several plant remedies used for the management of diabetes in Jamaica (Jones, 1955). In his study he evaluated the antidiabetic properties of bush teas from a wide variety of plants which include, periwinkle *(Vinca rosea)*, mistletoe *(Phthirusa pauciflora)*, nichol or nicker berry *(Coesalpinea bonducella)* and rice bitters *(Andrographis paniculata)* on 9 diabetic patients. From preliminary studies he found that the Nichol berry had no effect on either of the two patients treated; however two of the patients treated with periwinkle and one treated with mistletoe showed a significant decrease in glycosuria with a resulting decrease in blood glucose concentration. This response was very unusual; however Jones deduced that the increased blood glucose could have resulted from increasing reabsorption of sugar in the proximal renal tubules resulting in increases in the renal threshold of sugar in the body. Jones findings if accurate would indicate that such teas would prove harmful to diabetics and could potentially result in acute or chronic kidney disease.

In 1982, Morrison and West carried out preliminary investigations into the antidiabetic properties of several commonly used herbal remedies, using the Oral Glucose Tolerance Test (OGTT) in dogs. These plants included; bird pepper *(Capsicum frutescens)*, june plum *(Spondias dulcis)*, annatto *(Bixia orellana)*, guaco bush *(Mikania micrantha)*, cashew bark *(Anacardium occidentalis)*, cerasee *(Momordica charantia)*, periwinkle *(Catharanthus roseus)*, king of the forest *(Cassia alata)*, coconut *(Cocos nucifera)*, cumphrey *(Symphytum officinale)* and ganja *(Cannibis sativa)*. From their preliminary studies it was found that all plants except june plum and cannabis showed significant blood glucose lowering properties at some point during the test. Morrison and West further indicated that significant data were obtained to support the traditional use of annatto seed, bird pepper and periwinkle in diabetes management as the results obtained from the plant extracts indicated that they were able to sustain significant hypoglycemic effects in anesthetised dogs.

Further to these studies and the advent of easy access to advanced instrumentation researchers have been able to extract, isolate and identify the hypoglycemic principles and effectively test extracts from several herbal plants in Jamaica and the Caribbean both under in vitro and in vivo conditions. As such this chapter will highlight the scientific studies and antidiabetic principles present in the following plants; annatto *(Bixia orellana)*, bird pepper *(Capsicum frutescens)*, bitter yam *(Dioscorea polygonoides)*, dasheen *(Colocasia esculenta)*, cashew *(Anacardium occidentalis)*, cerasee *(Momordica charantia)*, periwinkle *(Catharanthus roseus)*, Pilea Elisabethae.

Based on the results from scientific studies it can be concluded that these eight (8) plants have significant potential for further scientific and clinical evaluations of the bioactive principles present. This may eventually result in one or more of these plants being developed as a useful drug for the management of Diabetes Mellitus.

However, despite the scientific evidence supporting the potential use of these plants in diabetes management, further scientific and clinical evaluations are required to determine their safety and efficacy before being use as alternative or complimentary remedies.

Bixa Orellana
(Annatto)

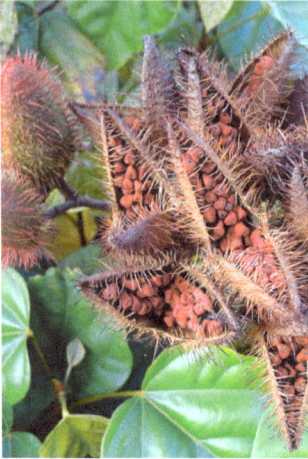

Botanical Classification

Kingdom:	Plantae
Order:	Malvales
Family:	Bixaceae
Genus:	Bixa
Species:	B. Orellana
Common Name:	Annato
Origin:	South America

Main Bioactives

Carotenoid (Trans-bixin-$C_{25}H_3O_4$), terpenes, bixin intermediates

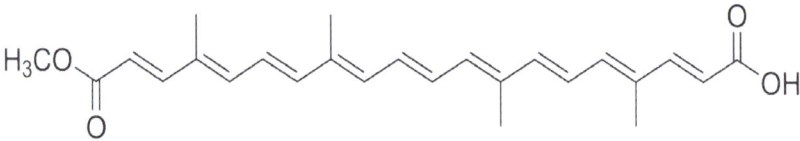

Figure 3: trans-bixin

The Annatto plant is a medium size shrub/small tree which grows between 2–3 metres in height. It is believed to have originated from Brazil and named after the Spanish conquistador, Francisco de Orellana, who is credited with discovering the Amazon River in 1541. The plant has a characteristic pink or white rose-like flower which after fertilization matures into a prickly reddish-orange heart-shaped pod with several seeds covered with a red aril. Trees are easy to cultivate, reaches maturity in 4–5 years and continue to bear up to 20 years. A single annatto tree can produce up to 270 kg of seeds per season, The annatto plant is commonly found in the Caribbean, South and Central America and some parts of Mexico.

Traditional Use

Jamaica once had a vibrant dye and food coloring industry

primarily sourced from the annatto plant. Before cheaper/ synthetic dyes were discovered, the annatto fruit was the number one choice for the production of yellow and red pigments predominantly used in foods, cosmetics and textile industries globally. It is predicted that this industry may become vibrant again owing to the rising demand for more natural plant-based food additives and dyes. Also there is an ointment developed from the annatto plant (Cumsee Ointment) that is used to treat leg ulcers. there is the observance of an Annatto festival in Jamaica in the town of Annotto Bay, St. Mary.

Scientific Studies

The diabetic properties of the plant were first studied by Morrison and West in 1982 (Morrison and West, 1982; 1985). Hyperglycemic (glucose raising) and hypoglycemic (glucose lowering) properties were reported upon oral administration of seed extracts to dogs at a dose of 400mg/kg body weight. Hyperglycemic properties were observed when the polar extract was administered and hypoglycemic properties when the non-polar extract was administered. Administration of the polar extract resulted in prolonged impaired glucose tolerance in dogs but not in rats. Thompson later isolated and purified the hyperglycemic compound, transbixin (Figure 3) from the extract. Pure transbixin, when administered to dogs resulted in hyperglycemic episodes and damage to the pancreas. Analysis of tissue samples revealed damage to mitochondria and endoplasmic reticulum mainly in liver and pancreas of the dogs treated (Morrison *et al.*, 1991). However, Thompson indicated that extracts used traditionally contained other components other than transbixin which could explain the positive properties experienced when consumed.

Russell *et al.* (2005) later developed a method to isolate the hypoglycemic principle from the crude extract which contained both hyperglycemic and hypogycemic principles. The hypoglycemic principle contained several compounds including terpenes and bixin intermediates. Russell *et al.* (2008) also reported that the mechanism of action of the hypoglycemic principle was similar to that of sulfonylureas, which are known diabetic hypoglycemic drugs. The extract acted by increasing the insulin levels, decreasing the glucagon levels, increasing the binding of insulin to its receptors, decreasing the levels of blood glucose and delaying the absorption of glucose from the gut. Russell *et al.* (2008) reported an 11 % reduction in blood glucose levels and 45 % increase in plasma insulin levels after 1 hour of administering the extract with hypoglycemic principles. Additionally, a 50 % increase in insulin affinity in mononuclear leucocytes and 92 % increase in erythrocytes were also reported.

Additionally, the effective dose was significantly reduced from the 400 mg/kg body weight previously reported by Morrison et al (1991) to 80 mg/kg body weight.

Capsicum Frutescens
(Bird Pepper)

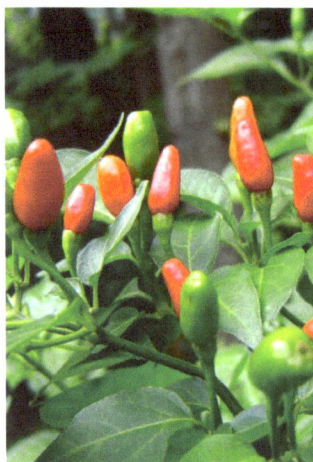

Botanical Classification

Kingdom:	Plantae
Order:	solanales
Family:	solanaceae
Genus:	capsicum
Species:	frutescens
Common Name:	Bird pepper
Origin:	Central America

Main Bioactive
Capsaicin ($C_{18}H_{27}NO_3$)

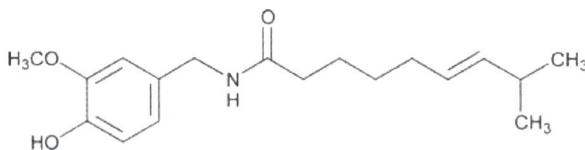

Figure 4: Capsaicin

Capsicum frutescens (bird pepper or Cayenne) is an annual short-lived perennial plant. Flowers are white with a greenish white or greenish yellow corolla, and are either insect or self-fertilized. The fruit typically grows in an erect position and are ellipsoid-conical to lanceoloid in shape. They are usually very small and pungent, growing 10–20 mm long and 3–7mm in diameter.

Geographical Location

Capsicum frutescens is believed to have originated in either South or Central America; however it grows widely in the tropics. The specie investigated in the Caribbean for anti-diabetic properties is commonly referred to as bird pepper and is found growing wild throughout Jamaica.

Traditional Usage

The fruits are traditionally used in the Caribbean to treat, the common cold, flu, hypertension, cardiovascular disease and diabetes.

Scientific Studies

Tolan *et al.* (1994) investigated the anti-diabetic properties of the fruit at the University of the West Indies, Mona. The researchers extracted the bioactive compound "capsaicin" from the fruit and investigated its effect on blood glucose, plasma insulin and insulin receptors in dogs with normal blood glucose levels. It was found that the dogs treated with capsaicin had a 23 % reduction in blood glucose concentration and 56 % increase in plasma insulin levels compared to the control group 2.5 hours after administering the bird pepper extract.

Tolan *et al.* (2001) also reported a significant reduction in percentage insulin receptor binding for the capsaicin treated dogs when compared with the control. A reduction of 73 % in insulin affinity and 70 % in insulin receptor sites were also reported. It is suggested that these reductions may be due to negative cooperativity which worked in conjunction with down-regulation. In other words, when one insulin molecule binds to the receptor site there is a reduction in the affinity for the binding of other insulin molecules.

The researchers concluded that capsaicin is the major constituent of Capsicum frutescens responsible for the hypoglycemic episodes observed in the dogs and that it also causes an increase in insulin secretion leading to a reduction in insulin binding on the insulin receptors along with decreases in insulin binding, insulin affinity and the amount of insulin receptor.

Tandan *et al.* (1991) also reported on the efficacy of capsicum based topical cream in treating diabetic neuropathy. In this study subjects were treated with a 0.075 % capsicum cream topically to treat diabetic neuropathy and intractable pain. Over 46 % of the participants reported pain relief during capsicum treatment with over 50% reporting improved pain control or complete cure compared to the control (23.2 %) at the end of the 8 week study.

Dioscorea Polygonoides
(Bitter Yam)

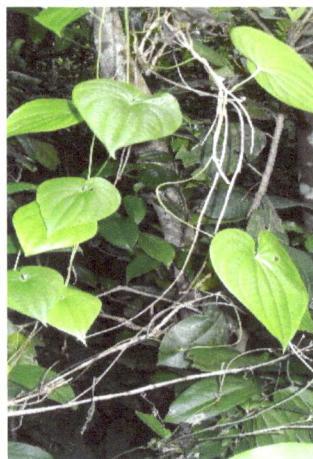

Botanical Classification

Kingdom:	Plantae
Order:	Liliales
Family:	Dioscoreaceae
Genus:	Dioscorea
Species:	Dioscorea polygonoides
Common Name:	Bitter Yam
Origin:	Africa

Main Bioactive

Diosgenin ($C_{27}H_{42}O_3$)

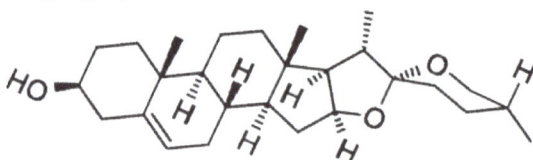

Figure 5: Diosgenin

Yams are angiosperms, or flowering plants. They are monocotyledons belonging to the family Dioscoreaceae within the order Dioscoreales. There are considerable variations in the size, shape and colour of the leaves and tubers. The leaves are often broad, heart-shaped with pellucid lines and may be smooth or hairy. The stem of the plant is rope-like in nature resulting in the plant being unable to stand on its own. Yams are primarily known for their high nutritional value with high carbohydrate-starch content (15–25%), protein (1–2.5%), fiber (0.5–1.5%), ash (0.7–2.0%) and fat (0.05–0.20 %). They are also known to be rich in vitamins and minerals along with other bioactive compounds such as cyanoglucosides, oxalate, phytic acid and phytosteroids.

Geographical Location

Yams are found in Africa (Nigeria, East Africa, South-East Asia), South America, Asia and the Caribbean region.

Traditional Usage

Yams are traditionally used as a food source and are listed as staple foods due to the high carbohydrate content of the tubers. In Jamaica, the bitter yam is traditionally used to make "roots tonic", eaten (after sun drying or roasting) and in some cultures as a contraceptive.

Scientific Studies

McAnuff-Harding et al (2006) reported on the hypoglycemic properties of a bitter yam extract. Three steroidal saponins (diosgenin, pennogenin, Delta-3 diosgenin) and two phytosterols (sitosterol and stigmasterol) were isolated and characterized. Over 80% of the extract contained diosgenin. In vivo studies carried out on streptozotocin induced diabetic and non-diabetic male wistar rats over a three week period confirmed diosgenin as the bioactive compound eliciting the primary hypoglycemic properties.

Studies on blood, intestinal and metabolic enzymes indicated that dietary supplementation with bitter yam sapogenin extract or commercial diosgenin significantly reduced disaccharidase activity. This is suggestive of lower levels of absorbable glucose from carbohydrate digestion leading to the reductions in blood glucose concentrations. It was also observed that bitter yam sapogenin extract significantly decreased fasting blood glucose concentration and Na^+-K^+-ATPase activity compared to the control group. Commercial diosgenin supplementation resulted in a significant increase in Ca2+ ATPase activity in proximal region compared to the diabetic control and bitter yam sapogenin extract groups.

The authors concluded that bitter yam sapogenin extract or commercial diosgenin action on intestinal Na^+-K^+-ATPase activity could account for their hypoglycemic properties. However, despite the potential benefits to diabetics, concerns were expressed regarding the significant decline in body weight. Uemura et al, (2010) reported that diosgenin ameliorated diabetes by promoting adipocyte differentiation and inhibiting inflammation in adipose tissues.

Colocasia Esculenta
(Dasheen)

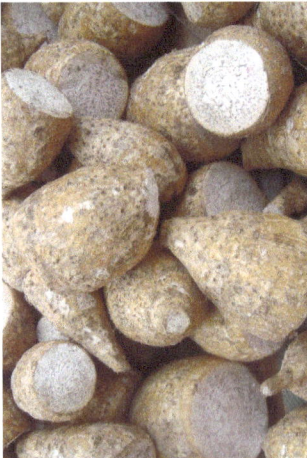

Botanical Classification

Kingdom:	*Plantae*
Order:	*Alismatales*
Family:	*Araceae*
Genus:	*Colocasia*
Species:	*Colocasia Esculenta*
Common Name:	*Dasheen*
Origin:	*Southeast Asia*

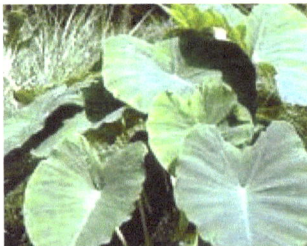

Main Bioactive

Linamarin ($C_{10}H_{17}NO_6$)

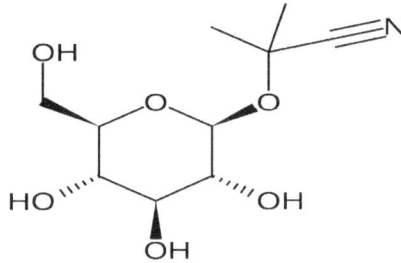

Figure 6: Linamarin

Dasheen is a perennial herbaceous monocotyledonous plant belonging to the Aracae family. The plant consists of a central corm from which the shoot, cormel and root arise. The shoot consists mainly of the leaves, which develop in a worl from the apex of the corm upwards. The leaves and shoot form the most prominent aerial part of the plant. The uncooked corm and leaves are believed to be toxic owing to the high levels of calcium oxalate (raphides). However, these are degraded after cooking or reduced after overnight steeping in cold water.

Geographical Location

The tubers are widely cultivated in subtropics and the tropical regions as a source of digestible carbohydrate. The plant is believed to have originated in Bangladesh and India and spread to the Caribbean and the Americas via Africa.

Traditional Use

The corm is consumed as a source of staple starch. The leaves and the petiole are used in Trinidad to make exotic stews referred to as "callaloo". The corms are usually roasted, baked or boiled while the leaves are steamed or stewed. The starch in the corm is easily digestible and as such is often used for baby food. The leaves are a good source of vitamins A and C and contain more protein than the corms and are believed to be a healing plant with various medicinal properties.

Scientific Studies

Grindley et al. (2001) extracted linamarin from Dioscorea Cayenensis (yam) and Colocasia esculenta (dasheen). The linamarin extracts were fed in conjunction with rodent feed to streptozotocin induced diabetic rats for four weeks. The effect of the plant liniamarin extracts were compared to commercial linamarin and non-diabetic and diabetic rats fed rodent feed only.

After four weeks of treatment, the results indicated that administration of commercial linamarin to diabetic rats led to a 7% increase in blood glucose concentrations compared to the diabetic control. Interestingly, administration of dasheen plant extract resulted in a 32% decrease in the blood glucose concentrations when compared to the diabetic control. The researchers suggest that the mechanism of action was not conclusive but could be due to the intestinal peripheral utilization of glucose. He also suggested that the soluble fibre present in the dasheen was a contributory factor in the hypoglycemic effect. These extracts also slightly lowered blood cholesterol, which is also important to diabetics.

Additionally, the researchers reported a significant increase in blood glucose concentration when commercial linamarin and the dasheen extract were administered to protein malnourished diabetic rats. The researchers concluded that the extract may be useful in lowering blood glucose concentrations; however it appeared that the extract also aggravated kidney damage induced by diabetes. As such, further work must be done on the extracts to identify the bioactive compounds that elicited the various effects observed.

Anacardium Occidentalis
(Cashew)

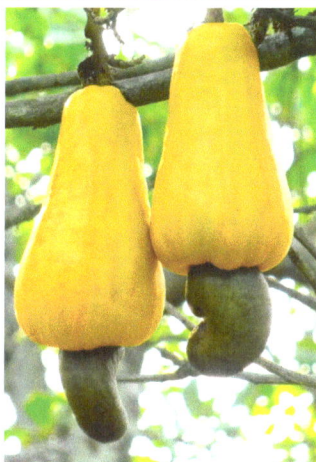

Botanical Classification

Kingdom:	Plantae
Order:	Sapindales
Family:	Anacardiaceae
Genus:	Anacardium
Species:	A. occidentale
Common Name:	Cashew
Origin:	South America

Main Bioactives

Phytosterols (stigmast-4-en-3-one [$C_{29}H_{48}O$] and stigmast-4-en-3-ol [$C_{29}H_{50}O$])

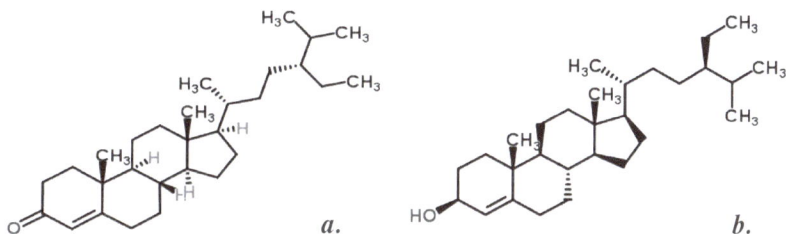

Figure 7: stigmast-4-en-3-one (a) and stigmast-4-en-3-ol (b)

Geographical Location

The evergreen tree is a part of the vegetation typical of the tropical countries of the world. Cashew is native plant to tropical America and the West Indies. It was brought to the region by the Portuguese and Spanish adventurers. The crop can be found growing throughout Jamaica but is mainly cultivated in St. Thomas, St. Catherine, Clarendon and St. Elizabeth.

Traditional Use

The bark is traditionally used as a treatment for diabetes mellitus. The pear-shaped fruit is used in various products such as juice, jam, syrup, chutney and beverage while the nuts are eaten raw or roasted.

Scientific Studies

Alexander-Lindo et al. (2004) extracted, isolated and purified the hypoglycemic principles from the bark of the cashew plant and studied its effect on blood glucose concentration in dogs. Analysis of the bioactives in the extracts revealed that they were steroidal in nature and belonged to the group of phytosterols. The researchers deduced that the compounds could have been formed from the auto-oxidation of β-sitosterol. They were then identified to be stigmast-4-en-3-ol and stigmast-4-en-3-one. The alcohol (stigmast-4-en-3-ol) is easily oxidized to the ketone (stigmast-4-en-3-one). The compounds were found to significantly reduce the blood glucose concentration of the test animals when the hexane extract of the tree bark was administered at a concentration of 300 mg/kg body weight (Alexander-Lindo et al. 2007). It is believed that the hypoglycemic and the synergistic effect of both compounds are responsible for the extracts hypoglycemic effect.

Additionally, stigmast-4-en-3-one was shown to be present in two enantiomeric forms in the mixture administered (90% in the + ve and 10% in the -ve form). The −ve form is rare and is also postulated to improve the blood glucose lowering effect of the compounds. The researchers postulated that stigmast-4-en-3-one causes an increase in the binding effect of insulin for its receptor, as a result of the presence of the ethyl group on the side chain. They also suggested that the compounds induced delayed absorption of glucose similar to α-glucosidase inhibitors with a possible mode of action similar to the sulphonylurea glibenclamide.

Catharanthus Roseus
(Periwinkle)

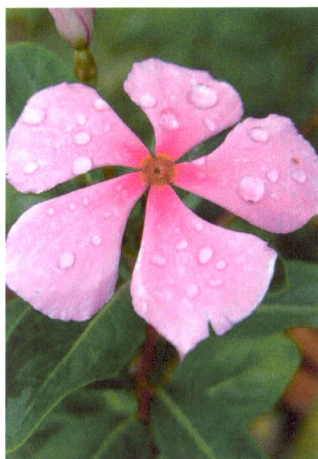

Botanical Classification

Kingdom:	*Plantae*
Order:	*Gentianales*
Family:	*Apocynaceae*
Genus:	*Catharanthus*
Species:	*C. Roseus*
Common Name:	*Periwinkle*
Origin:	*West Indies*

Main Bioactives

Alkaloids (catharanthine, leurosine sulphate, lochnerine, tetrahydroalstonine, vindoline and vindolinine)

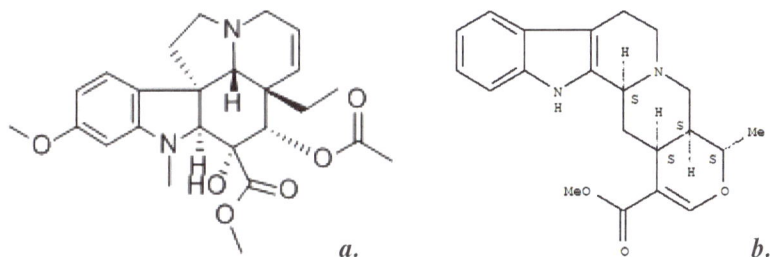

Figure 8. vindoline (a) and tetrahydroalstonine (b)

Geographical Location

Periwinkle is a bushy perennial herb belonging to the Apocynaceae family. The plants usually grow up to 75 cm in height and may possess white, crimson or lavender-pink flowers. The plant is native to the West Indies and can be found growing widely in tropical and subtropical regions.

Traditional use

Periwinkle is normally used for the treatment of hypertension and cancer but is primarily consumed in the West Indies as a treatment for diabetes. The leaves, roots, stem and flowers are usually boiled in water to produce a tea for oral consumption. In folklore medicine it is believed that consumption of five leaves, three times per day as a hot beverage is enough to manage blood glucose levels in diabetics.

Scientific Studies

The hypoglycemic properties of periwinkle have been extensively studied and have been shown to be effective in the treatment of diabetes. Banakar et al (2007) reported a 6.5-12% decrease in postprandial blood glucose in diabetic males and females treated with 2 g dried leaves per day for 1 month. Additionally, a 2% reduction in total cholesterol, 4% in triglycerides and 3% reduction in LDL were also reported. Benjamin et al (1994) also reported a reduction in serum glucose of 60 % after administration of water extracts intragastrically to male streptozotocin induced diabetic rats.

Additionally, Jayanthi et al (2010) reported a decrease in serum glucose concentration of 54% upon administration of 200mg/kg body weight of a dichlormethane/methanol extract to alloxan induced diabetic rats. A corresponding 40% reduction in blood urea and 28% in total cholesterol was also reported after administration of the extract over a 20-day period. It is believed that alkaloids present in the plant such as catharanthine, leurosine sulphate, lochnerine, tetrahydroalstonine, vindoline and vindolinine are responsible for the hypoglycemic properties.

Nammi et al (2003) reported that *C. roseus* produced dose-dependent reduction in blood glucose of both normal and diabetic rabbits which were comparable to that of the sulfonylurea glibenclamide. They further stated that the extracts resulted in a prolonged action in reduction of blood glucose. Owing to this it is believed that the proposed mechanism of action of the hypoglycemic principles involves reduction in enzymic activities of glycogen synthase, glucose 6-phosphate-dehydrogenase, succinate dehydrogenase and malate dehydrogenase resulting in increased glucose metabolism and enhancement of insulin secretion from the beta-cells of Langerhans or through extrapancreatic mechanism.

Pilea Elizabethae
(Pillea)

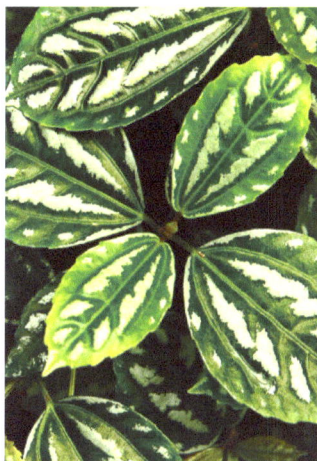

Botanical Classification

Kingdom:	Plantae
Order:	Rosidae
Family:	Urticaceae
Genus:	Pilea
Species:	P. elizabethae
Common Name:	Pillea
Origin:	

Main Bioactives

Beta-sitosterol and oleanonic acid

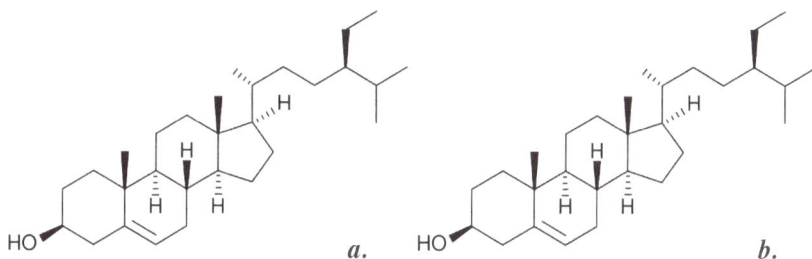

Figure 9. β-sitosterol (a) and oleanonic acid (b)

Pilea Elizabethae is a variety of the American botanical Pilea otherwise known as the aluminum plant. It is usually found growing wildly in the hilly, limestone regions of Jamaica and was first identified in St. Elizabeth by the Jamaican botanist, C.D. Adams in 1972.

Traditional use

The leaves of the plant are traditionally used to treat diabetes and other illnesses

Scientific Studies

Salmon and Lindo (2007) investigated the hypoglycemic properties of Pilea on normogluco Wistar rats. The data indicated significant reduction in blood glucose concentrations resulting from the bioactivity of both beta-sitosterol (phytosterol) and oleanonic acid (triterpenoid). Both compounds were previously shown to possess anti-flammatory properties; however hypoglycemic properties were not investigated. Interestingly, the hypoglycemic activity of the extract was most effective when both compounds were administered together, thereby indicating a synergistic relationship. They were identified as short-acting compounds which could be useful in reducing the risk or managing hypoglycemic episodes.

Momordica charantia L.
(Cerasee)

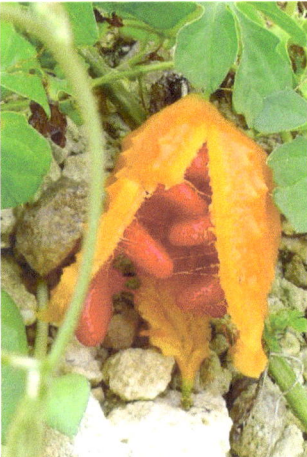

Botanical Classification

Kingdom:	Plantae
Order:	Violales
Family:	Cucurbitaceae
Genus:	Momordica
Species:	M. Charantia L
Common Name:	Cerasee
Origin:	Africa and Middle East

Main Bioactives
Mormordicin, Polypeptide-p and Charantin (stearoidal saponin)

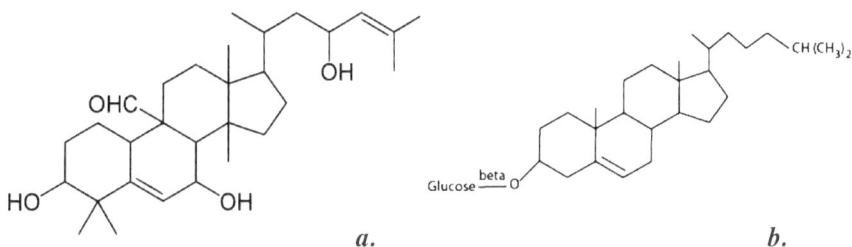

a.   *b.*

Figure 10. momordicin (a) and charantin (b)

Cerasee, a wild variety of Momordica charantia belongs to the family Cucurbitaceae and grows widely in tropical and subtropical regions, including parts of the Amazon Basin, Africa, Asia, the Caribbean and South America. The plant grows as a vine with green leaves, yellow flowers oblong green fruits (orange when ripe with bright red seeds.

Traditional use

Cerasee is traditionally prepared as a tea and consumed as a tonic, general prophylactic and in the treatment of diabetes mellitus in the West Indies and Central America. The leaves and stem are usually boiled and served as tea either sweetened or unsweetened.

Scientific Studies

Bailey et al (1985) investigated the hypoglycemic properties of cerasee in normal and stretozotocin induced rats. Intraperitoneal administration of an aqueous extract in normal mice, resulted in significant improvements in glucose tolerance after 8 hr, and a reduction in the level of hyperglycemia by 50% in streptozotocin diabetic mice after 5 hr. Chronic oral administration of cerasee extract to normal mice for 13 days also showed significant improvements in glucose tolerance. Unlike its close relative, bitter melon it did not significantly alter plasma insulin concentrations, thus suggesting that cerasee may exert an extrapancreatic effect to promote glucose disposal.

The hypoglycemic principles in cerasee and bitter melon have been attributed to the presence and action of momordicin, polypeptide-p and charantin. Bitter melon (cerasee's cousin) has been widely studied and shown to possess good antidiabetic properties. The hypoglycemic principles are believed to result in decreased hepatic gluconeogenesis, increased hepatic glycogen synthesis, increased peripheral glucose oxidation in erythrocytes and adipocytes and increased pancreatic insulin secretion (Shibib et al 1993; Welihinda *et al* 1982).

Despite the presence of overwhelming scientific data on *Mormordica charantia* (bitter melon) in the management of diabetes mellitus and its closeness to cerasee, additional work is required to further investigate cerasee's hypoglycemic properties. Additionally, such studies should investigate the possible mechanism of action of its bioactives, the effective dosage and evaluations on toxicity and safety.

References

Alexander-Lindo R., Morrison E.Y., Nair G.2004. 'Hypoglycemic effect of stigmast-4-en-3-one and its corresponding alcohol from the bark of Anacardium occidentale (cashew)'. Phytotherapy Research, no. 18(5):403-7.

Alexander-Lindo R., Morrison E.Y., et al. 2007. 'Effect of the Fractions of the Hexane Bark Extract and Stigmast-4-en-3-one Isolated from Anacardium occidentale on Blood Glucose Tolerance Test in an Animal Model'. International. Journal of Pharmacology, no.3 (1): 41-47.

Bachrach,U. and Yaniv, Z. 2005.Handbook of Medicinal Plants. Food Products Press and The Haworth Press Inc.

Bailey CJ, Day C, Turner SL, Leatherdale BA.1985. 'Cerasee, a traditional treatment for diabetes. Studies in normal and streptozotocin diabetic mice'. Diabetes Research, no.2:81-4.

Banakar V, Malagi U., and Naik R .2007.' Impact of Periwinkle Leaves (Catharanthus roseus) on Management of Diabetes Mellitus'. Karnataka Journal of Agricultural Sciences, no.20: 115 – 119.

Benjamin BD, Kelkar SM, Pote MS, et al.1994. 'Catharanthus roseus cell culture: Growth, alkaloid synthesis and antidiabetic activity'. Phytotherapy Research, no. 8(3): 185-186.

Grindley, P. B., Omoruyi, Felix O., et al.2001.' Blood lipids and lipid metabolism in the liver of sreptozotocin-induced diabetic rats fed organic extracts of yam (d. cayenensis, cv. round leaf yellow yam) and dasheen (c. esculenta)'. International Journal of Food, Sciences and Nutrition. no.52: 429-33.

Jayanthi, M., Sowbala, N., et al. 2010. 'A study of anti-hyperglycemic effect of Catharanthus roseus in alloxan induced diabetic rats'. International Journal of Pharmacy and Pharmaceutical Sciences, no.2 (4). 114116

Jones H. P. 1995. Diabetes in Jamaica. Lancet. 891-897.

McAnuff MA., Harding WW., et al. 2005. 'Hypoglycemic effects of steroidal sapogenins isolated from Jamaican bitter yam, Dioscorea polygonoides'. Food and Chemical Toxicology, no. 43 (11):1667-1672

Mitchell, S. and Ahmad, M. H. 1948-2001. 'A Review of Medicinal Plant Research at the University of the West Indies Jamaica'. West Indian Medical Journal vol. 55, no.4.

Morrison, E.Y. and Thompson, H. 1991. 'Extraction of an hyperglycemic principle from the annatto (Bixa orellana); a medicinal plant in the West Indies'. Tropical and Geographical Medicine, no. 43(1-2):184-188.

Morrison E.Y and West M.E. 1982. 'A preliminary study of the effects of some West Indian medicinal plants on blood sugar levels in the dog'. West Indian Medical Journal, no. 31: 194-197

Morrison E.Y and West M.E. 1985. 'The effect of Bixa orellana (annatto) on blood sugar levels in the anaesthetized dog'. West Indian Medical Journal, no. 34: 38-42.

Nammi, S and Boini, M.K. 2003. 'The juice of fresh leaves of Catharanthus Roseus Linn. Reduces blood glucose in normal and alloxan diabetic rabbits'. BMC Complementary and Alternative Medicine, no.3:4.

Oliver-Bever, B. Oral hypoglycemic action of medicinal plants in tropical West Africa. Cambridge University Press, 1986.

Russell, K.R., Morrison E.Y., Ragoobirsingh D. 2005. 'The effect of annatto on insulin binding properties in the dog'. Phytotherapy Research, no.19 (5): 433-436.

Russell K.R and Omoruyi F.O. 2008. 'Hypoglycemic activity of Bixa orellana extract in the dog'. Methods and Findings in Experimental and Clinical Pharmacology, no.30 (4): 301-5.

Shibib B.A., Khan L.A., Rahman R. 1993. 'Hypoglycemic activity of Coccinia indica and Momordica charantia in diabetic rats: depression of the hepatic gluconeogenetic enzymes glucose-6-phosphatase and fructose-1,6-biphosphatase and elevation of both liver and red cell shunt enzyme glucose-6-phosphate dehydrogenase'. Biochemical Journal, No.(292): 267-70.

Singh S.N. and Vats P. et al. 2001 'Effect of an antidiabetic extract of Catharanthus roseus on enzymic activities in streptozotocin induced diabetic rats'. Journal of Ethnopharmacology, no. (3):269-77

Tandan P. and Lewis G.A. 1991. 'Topical Capsaicin in Painful Diabetic Neuropathy: Controlled Study With Long-Term Follow-Up'. Diabetes Care, no.15 (1): 8-14

Tolan I., Ragoobirsingh D., and Morrison E.Y. 2004. 'Isolation and Purification of the Hypoglycemic Principle Present in Capsicum frutescens'. Phytotherapy Research, no. 18(1): 95-96.

Tolan I., Ragoobirsingh D., Morrison EY. 2001. 'The effect of capsaicin on blood glucose, plasma insulin levels and insulin binding in dog models'. Phytotherapy Research, no.15:391-394

Uemura T. and Hirai S. 2010. 'Diosgenin present in fenugreek improves glucose metabolism by promoting adipocyte differentiation and inhibiting inflammation in adipose tissues'. Molecular Nutrition and Food Research, no. 54 (11):1596-608.

Welihinda J. and Arvidson G. et al. 1982.'The insulin-releasing activity of the tropical plant Momordica charantia'. Acta Biologica et Medica Germanica, no.41: 1229-40.

WHO Expert Committee on Diabetes mellitus.1980. 'Technical report series 646'. World Health Organization.

4 Plants suspected to have Anti-Diabetic Properties based on Folklore

This section looks at commonly used plants, based on folklore medicine, for the treatment and management of diabetes. Little or no scientific information on their bioactive principles or usefulness to treat diabetes is available. Nevertheless, they form a significant part of the ethno-medicinal treatment of the disease and therefore cannot be ignored. In fact, more scientific studies need to be done to determine efficacy and toxicity as soon as possible in order to determine their potential for producing possible drug candidates.

It should also be noted that the uses of these folkloric herbal remedies have increased considerably and have gained high reputation in treating diabetes and it complications. In low socio-economic groups these herbal remedies are usually the first choice for treatment over conventional medicines.

The parts of the plants used vary from the leaves, stems, roots and in some cases the whole plant is used according to traditional practices. For some plants their uses are restricted geographically to individual or multiple Caribbean countries while others are used throughout the region. However, before making a final decision about the use of herbal remedies, it is best to know the advantages and disadvantages of these herbal medicines. This is to ensure that the plant selected for use will address the specified health related concern and will have little or no toxic effect or any other adverse side effects.

Despite the popular folklore use of a particular plant for treating diabetes and although "word of mouth recommendations have been given for these plants" extreme caution should be exercised in accepting these recommendations. Individuals are been reminded that these particular plants referred to in this section

have little or no scientific validation as been useful for diabetes management and therefore until new evidence emerges these plants should not be used in this regard.

The following is the list of plants used as Anti-diabetic medicinal agents which are based essentially on folklore and have had little or no scientific evaluation:

Aloe Vera
Common Name: Sinkle Bible

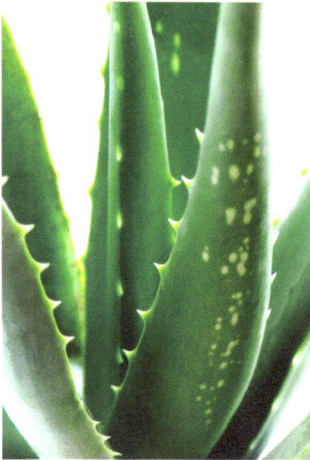

Botanical Classification

Kingdom:	Plantae
Order:	Liliales
Family:	Aloaceae
Genus:	Aloe
Species:	A. Vera

Origin: Africa

Traditional Use:
The Aloe leaf is put to soak in water and consumed as a drink to treat diabetes.

Allium Sativum

Common Name: *Garlic*

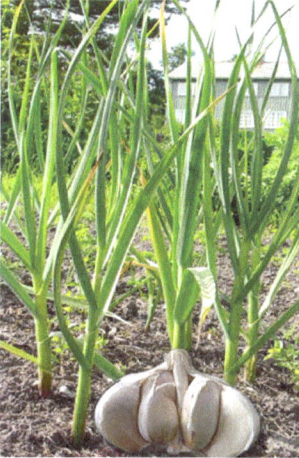

Botanical Classification

Kingdom:	Plantae
Order:	Liliales
Family:	Liliaceae
Genus:	Allium
Species:	A. Sativum

Origin: Central Asia

Traditional Use:

The root nodules are crushed and steeped in water and taken as a tonic.

Annona Muricata

Common Name: *Annona Muricata*

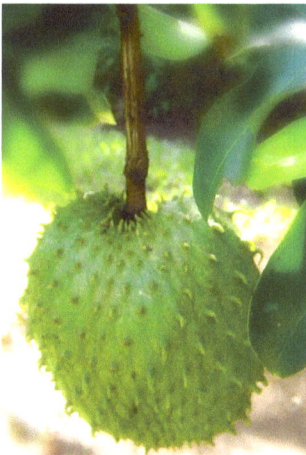

Botanical Classification

Kingdom:	Plantae
Order:	Magnoliales
Family:	Annonaceae
Genus:	Annona
Species:	A. Muricata

Origin: Mesoamerica

Traditional Use:

The bark and leaves of the soursop tree have been used traditionally in the Caribbean and in particular Jamaica to treat diabetes. Early studies have implied that these folkloric claims may be true since methanolic extracts of the leaves have shown to possess hypoglycemic properties (Jain et al, 2010).

Annona Squamosa
Common Name: *Sweetsop, Sugar Apple*

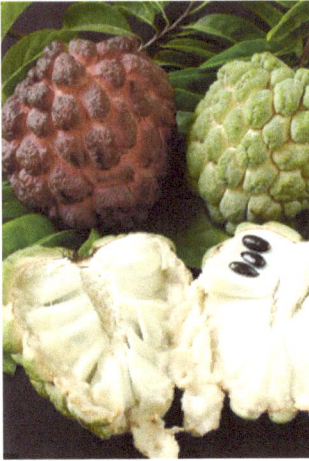

Botanical Classification

Kingdom:	Plantae
Order:	Magnoliales
Family:	Annonaceae
Genus:	Annona
Species:	A. Squamosa

Origin: unknown

Traditional Use:

The leaves are brewed to make tea.

Antigonon Leptopus
Common Name: *Chain of love*

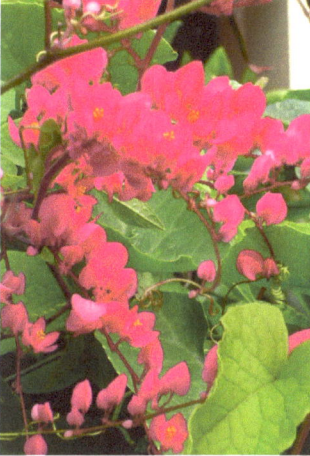

Botanical Classification

Kingdom:	Plantae
Order:	Polygonales
Family:	Polygonaceae
Genus:	Antigonon
Species:	A. Leptopus

Origin: Mexico

Traditional Use:

The exact part of plant used in folklore differs throughout the Caribbean islands. In Jamaica, the bright colorful flowers are sun dried and used to make tea.

Azadirachta Indica
Common Name: *Neem*

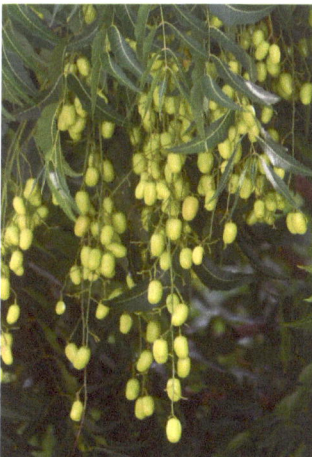

Botanical Classification

Kingdom:	Plantae
Order:	Sapindales
Family:	Meliaceae
Genus:	Azadircahta
Species:	A. Indica

Origin: India

Traditional Use:

A tea made from the leaves is used to treat diabetes. Early studies have hypothesized that extracts from the leaves as well as the fruit have shown to reduce insulin in blood (Ebong, 2008).

Bidens Alba
Common Name: *Butterfly Needles*

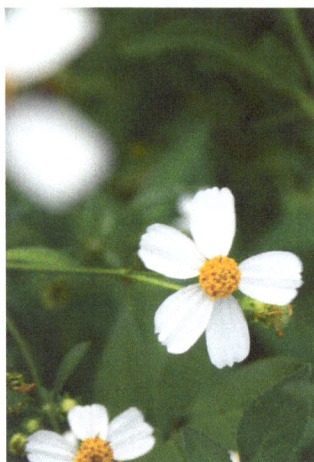

Botanical Classification

Kingdom:	Plantae
Order:	Asterales
Family:	Asteraceae
Genus:	Bidens
Species:	B. Alba

Origin: South America

Traditional Use:

The entire plant (leaves, stems, flowers and roots) is used in folklore medicine. They are brewed and consumed as a tea. Usually the flower is collected before it opens, rinsed, sun-dried then cut into pieces or compressed.

Bidens Pilosa
Common Name: *Spanish needle*

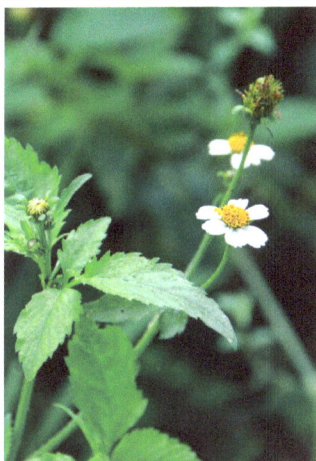

Botanical Classification

Kingdom:	Plantae
Order:	Asterales
Family:	Asteraceae
Genus:	Bidens
Species:	B. Pilosa

Origin: South America

Traditional Use:

The whole herb is used to make a tonic drink and used to lower blood sugar levels. It is suggested that the effect of the water extract of the plant on type 2 diabetes may aid in regulating insulin secretion and islet protection (Hsu et al., 2009).

Blighia Sapida
Common Name: *Ackee*

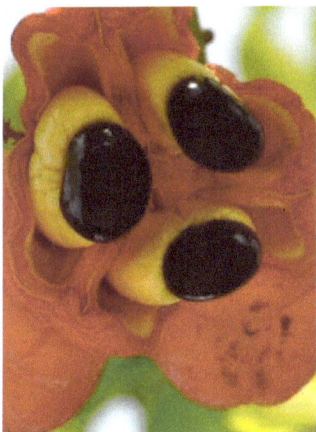

Botanical Classification

Kingdom:	Plantae
Order:	Sapindales
Family:	Sapindaceae
Genus:	Blighia
Species:	B. Sapida

Origin: West Africa

Traditional Use:

The fruit is boiled and eaten. Some scientists suggest that the fruit contains sterols which are believed to be capable of decreasing blood glucose rate (Olubunmi et al, 2009).

Bontia Daphnoides
Common Name: *Olive bush*

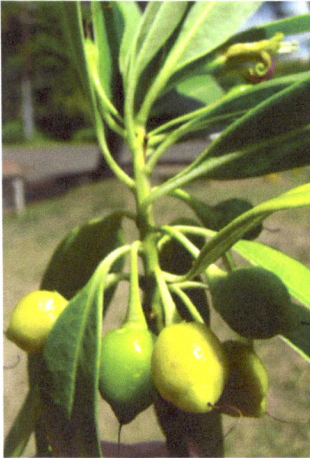

Botanical Classification

Kingdom:	Plantae
Order:	Scrophulariales
Family:	Myoporaceae
Genus:	Bontia
Species:	B. Daphnoides

Origin: Australia

Traditional Use:

The leaves and fruit are used traditionally to treat diabetic symptoms.

Caesalpinia Bonducella
Common Name: *Grey Nicker*

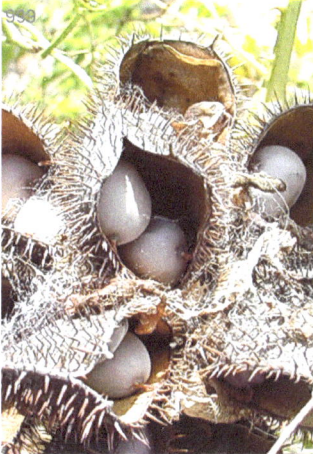

Botanical Classification

Kingdom:	Plantae
Order:	Fabales
Family:	Fabaceae
Genus:	Caesalpinia
Species:	C. Bonducella

Origin: Africa

Traditional Use:

The seeds are primarily used to make tea. They are prepared first by drying then grounded and brewed.

Capsicum Baccatum
Common Name: *Hot Pepper*

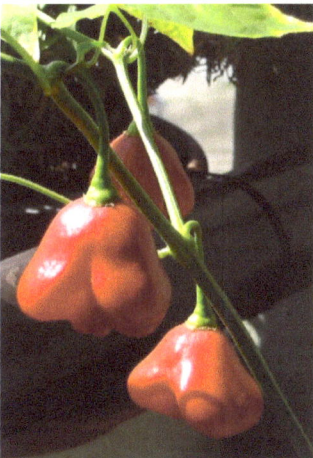

Botanical Classification

Kingdom:	Plantae
Order:	Solanales
Family:	Solanaceae
Genus:	Capsicum
Species:	C. Baccatum

Origin: Bolivia or Peru

Traditional Use:

The portion of the plant used traditionally is the fruit (pepper).

Carica Papaya L.
Common Name: *Papaya*

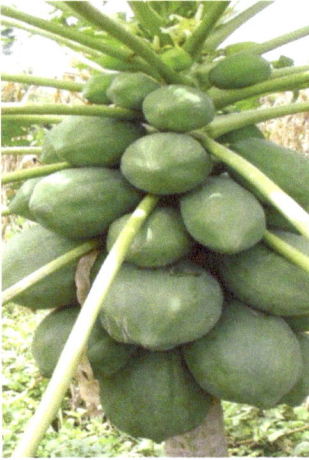

Botanical Classification

Kingdom:	Plantae
Order:	Violales
Family:	Caricaceae
Genus:	Carica
Species:	C. Papaya

Origin: Tropical Americas

Traditional Use:

The leaves of the plant are used to make tea to help with lowering blood glucose levels.

Cassia Alata
Common Name: *King of the forest*

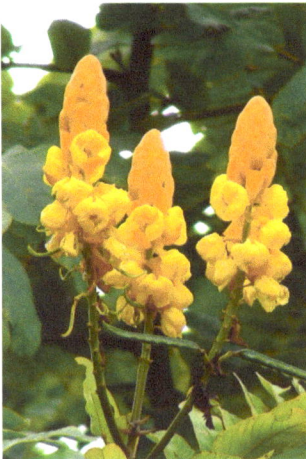

Botanical Classification

Kingdom:	Plantae
Order:	Fabales
Family:	Fabaceae
Genus:	Senna
Species:	S. Alata

Origin: South America

Traditional Use:

The portion of the plant used traditionally differs through the

Caribbean. However, the leaf is most widely used in Jamaica. Some preliminary scientific studies by Palanichamy in 1988 suggested that the leaves may seem to possess hypoglycemic (lowering of blood sugar levels) properties

Cassia Occidentalis
Common Name: Dandelion

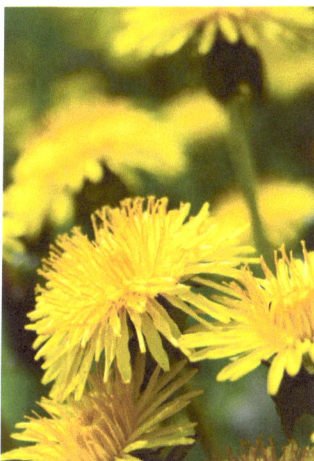

Botanical Classification

Kingdom:	Plantae
Order:	Fabales
Family:	Fabaceae
Genus:	Cassia
Species:	C. Occidentalis

Origin: Tropical America

Traditional Use:

The petals are dried and used in making tea. Preliminary research suggests that the plant contains triterpenes which are believed to have anti-diabetic property and responsible for stimulating insulin release (Verma et al, 2010).

Cecropia Peltata
Common Name: Embauba

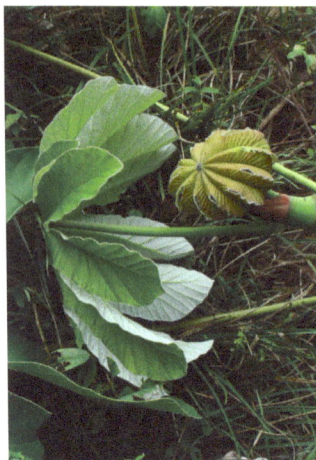

Botanical Classification

Kingdom:	Plantae
Order:	Urticales
Family:	Cecropiaceae
Genus:	Cecropia
Species:	C. Peltata

Origin: Central America

Traditional Use:

The leaves are used in Guatemala and Mexico to reduce blood sugar levels when consumed as a tea.

Chichorium Intybus
Common Name: Chicory or Endive

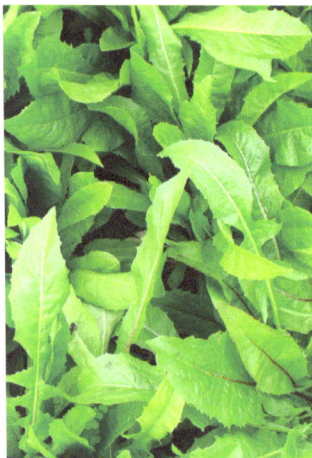

Botanical Classification

Kingdom:	Plantae
Order:	Asterales
Family:	Asteraceae
Genus:	Cichorium
Species:	C. Intybus

Origin: India

Traditional Use:

The leaves of the plant are used to make tea to help with lowering blood glucose levels.

Cocos Nucifera
Common Name: *Coconut*

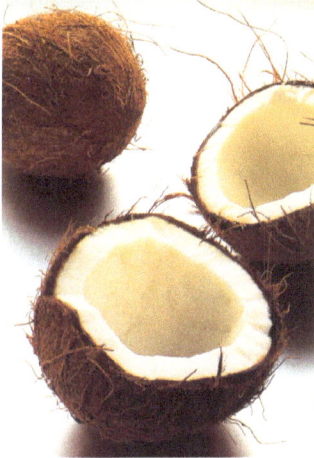

Botanical Classification

Kingdom:	Plantae
Order:	Arecales
Family:	Arecaceae
Genus:	Cosos
Species:	C. Nucifera

Origin: Asian Peninsular

Traditional Use:

The coconut husk (shell) and pulp of the fruit is commonly used by diabetics. The coconut water is rich in nutrients and also aid in lowering blood sugar levels. It is believed by some scientists to improve insulin secretion which leads to lowering of blood sugar levels.

Cuminum Cyminum
Common Name: *Cumin seeds*

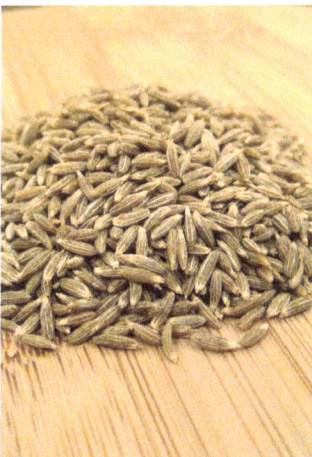

Botanical Classification

Kingdom:	Plantae
Order:	Apiales
Family:	Apiaceae
Genus:	Cuminum
Species:	C. Cyminum

Origin: Western Asia

Traditional Use:

The seeds are eaten raw to lower blood sugar levels.

Curcuma Longa
Common Name: Turmeric

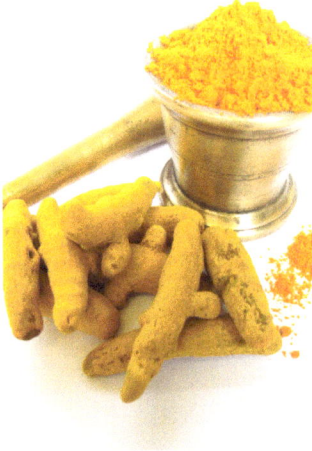

Botanical Classification

Kingdom:	Plantae
Order:	Zingiberales
Family:	Zingiberaceae
Genus:	Curcuma
Species:	C. Longa

Origin: India

Traditional Use:

In folklore, two full tea spoons taken with each meal reduces blood sugar as well as secondary symptoms that may accompany diabetes such as hyperlipidemia.

Gomphrena Globosa
Common Name: *Bachelor button*

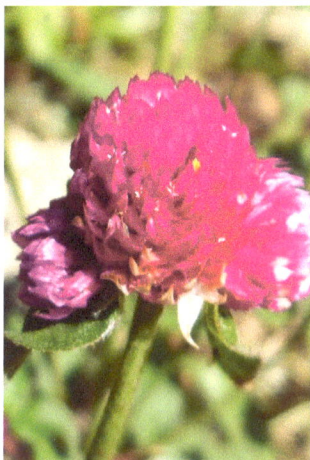

Botanical Classification

Kingdom:	Plantae
Order:	Caryophyllales
Family:	Amaranthaceae
Genus:	Gomphrena
Species:	G. Globosa

Origin: China

Traditional Use:

The flowers are commonly used by diabetics. Firstly the flowers are picked, washed and sun dried. They are then brewed to make tea which is said to have a pleasant aroma.

Ganoderma Lucidum
Common Name: *Reishi mushroom*

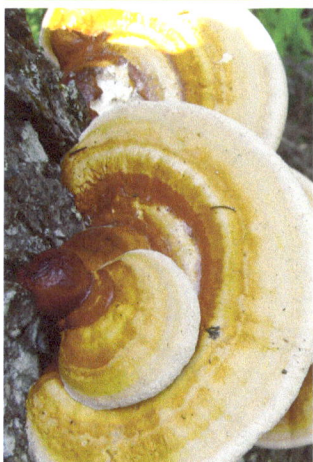

Botanical Classification

Kingdom:	Fungi
Order:	Polyporales
Family:	Ganodermataceae
Genus:	Ganoderma
Species:	G. Lucidum

Origin: Asia

Traditional Use:

The plant is found in the Caribbean and South America. It is used to maintain blood sugar levels as well as to prevent complications caused by diabetes. The mushroom is dried, milled and used as a tea.

Hibiscus Sabdariffa
Common Name: Sorrel

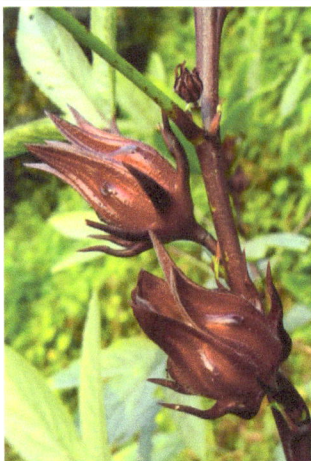

Botanical Classification

Kingdom:	Plantae
Order:	Malvales
Family:	Malvaceae
Genus:	Hibiscus
Species:	H. Sabdariffa

Origin: Egypt

Traditional Use:

Sorrel drink is very popular in Jamaica and the Caribbean. The sorrel fruit is rich in anti-oxidants that prevent the cells in the body from oxidative stress. The sorrel is steeped in warm water and consumed unsweetened by diabetics who reported that it lowers sugar levels and hypertension.

Lepidium Meyenii
Common Name: *Maca root*

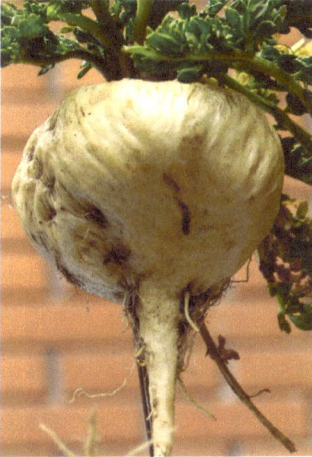

Botanical Classification

Kingdom:	Plantae
Order:	Capparales
Family:	Brassicaceae
Genus:	Lepidium
Species:	L. Meyenii

Origin: Unknown

Traditional Use:

The plant roots and leaves have been noted to possess some anti-diabetic properties.

Luffa Acutangula
Common Name: *Turai*

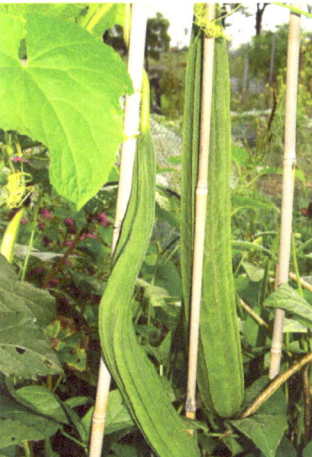

Botanical Classification

Kingdom:	Plantae
Order:	Violales
Family:	Cucurbitaceae
Genus:	Luffa
Species:	L. Acutanfula

Origin: India

Traditional Use:

This plant is found in Guadeloupe, Antigua, Dominica, St. Vincent and Martinique. The leaves and fruit are dried and used in tea preparations.

Mikania Micrantha
Common Name: *Guaco*

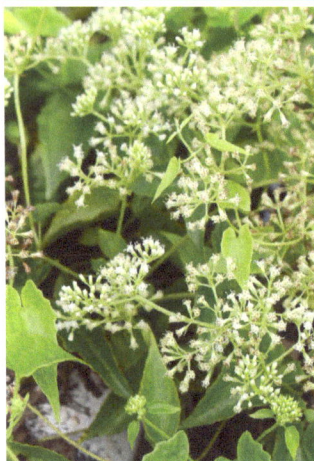

Botanical Classification

Kingdom:	Plantae
Order:	Asterales
Family:	Asteraceae
Genus:	Mikania
Species:	Mikania Micrantha

Origin: South America

Traditional Use:

The leaves are traditionally used as a tea.

Neurolaena Lobata
Common Name: *Jackass bitters*

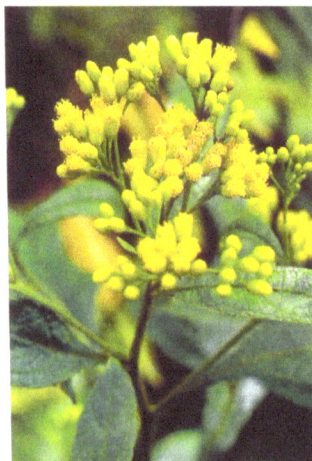

Botanical Classification

Kingdom:	Plantae
Order:	Asterales
Family:	Asteraceae
Genus:	Neurolaena
Species:	N. Lobata

Origin: Unknown

Traditional Use:

The leaves of the plant are used to make tea to help with lowering blood glucose levels.

Opuntia Streptacantha
Lemaire
Common Name: *Nopal cactus or Prickly pear cactus*

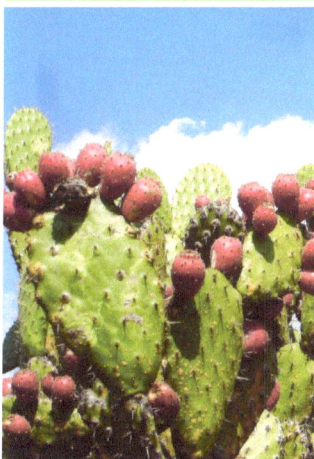

Botanical Classification

Kingdom:	Plantae
Order:	Caryophyllales
Family:	Cactaceae
Genus:	Opuntia
Species:	O. Streptacantha

Origin: Africa

Traditional Use:

The plant has been used in the Caribbean and South America as a medicinal plant. Both the sap and the leaves have been suggested to have positive effects on postprandial glucose levels in type 2 individuals.

Psidium Guajava
Common Name: Guava

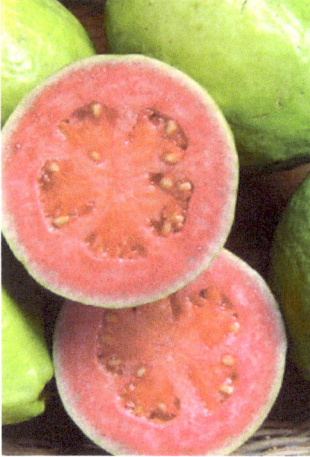

Botanical Classification

Kingdom:	Plantae
Order:	Myrtales
Family:	Myrtaceae
Genus:	Psidium
Species:	P. Guajava

Origin: Tropical America

Traditional Use:

The fruit is believed to contain anti-oxidants and helpful towards persons with diabetes.

Phyllanthus Amarus
Common Name: Button-under-leaf or Seed-under-leaf

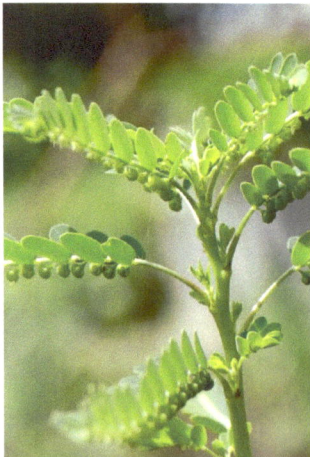

Botanical Classification

Kingdom:	Plantae
Order:	Malpighiales
Family:	Phyllanthaceae
Genus:	Phyllanthus
Species:	P. Amarus

Origin: Nigeria

Traditional Use:

The leaves are traditionally used as a tea.

Solanum Lycopersicum
Common Name: *Tomato*

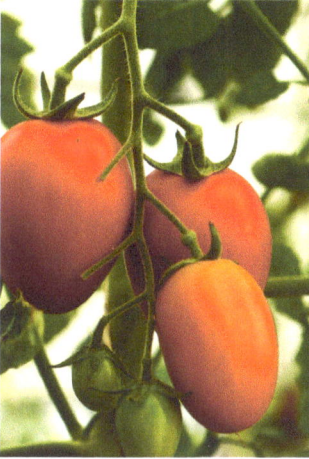

Botanical Classification

Kingdom:	Plantae
Order:	Solanales
Family:	Solanaceae
Genus:	Solanum
Species:	S. Lycopersicum

Origin: unknown

Traditional Use:

The fruit is consumed and reports have indicated that it contains malic acid which may be capable of stimulating insulin release.

Silybum Marianum
Common Name: *Milk thistle*

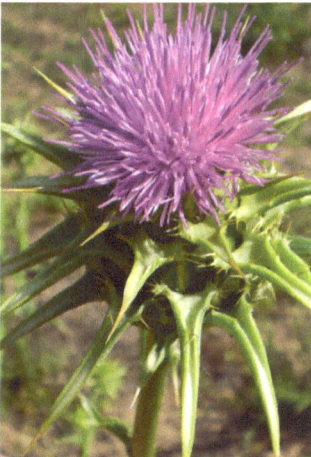

Botanical Classification

Kingdom:	Plantae
Order:	Asterales
Family:	Asteraceae
Genus:	Silybum
Species:	S. Marianum

Origin: Southern Europe

Traditional Use:

The flowers are dried and used to make tea.

Spondias Dulcis
Common Name: June plum

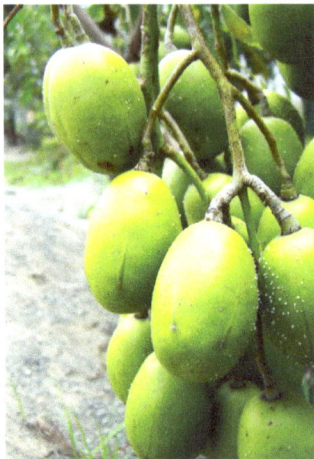

Botanical Classification

Kingdom:	Plantae
Order:	Sapindales
Family:	Anacardiaceae
Genus:	Spondias
Species:	Spondias Dulcis

Origin: Melanesia

Traditional Use:

The leaves and fruit have been claimed to manage diabetes and its symptoms. The leaves are used to make tea and the fruits are consumed green.

Symphytum Officinale
Common Name: Comfrey

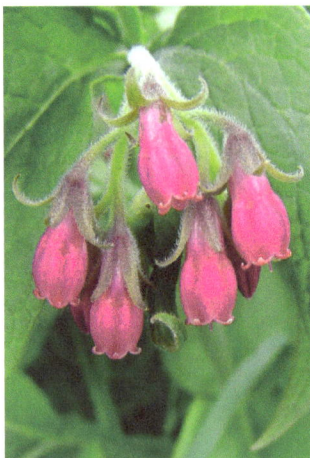

Botanical Classification

Kingdom:	Plantae
Order:	Lamiales
Family:	Boraginaceae
Genus:	Symphytum
Species:	S. Offinale

Origin: Europe

Traditional Use:

The portions of the plant used traditionally are the dried petals for making tea.

Trigonella Foenu-Greacum
Common Name: Fenugreek

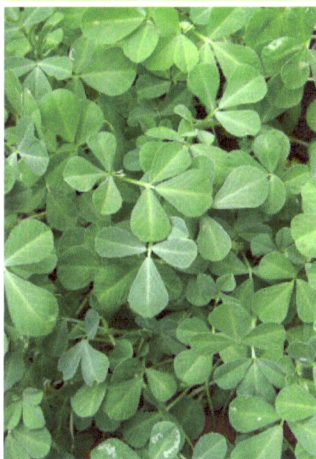

Botanical Classification

Kingdom:	Plantae
Order:	Fabales
Family:	Fabaceae
Genus:	Trigonella
Species:	T. Foenum-Graecum

Origin: Mediterranean

Traditional Use:

The leaves are dried and used to make tea. Preliminary studies reported that the leaves contain the amino acid, 4-hydroxyisoleucine which stimulate insulin secretion and may help with lowering blood sugar levels (Mitra, 2006).

Tunera Diffusa
Common Name: **Damiana**

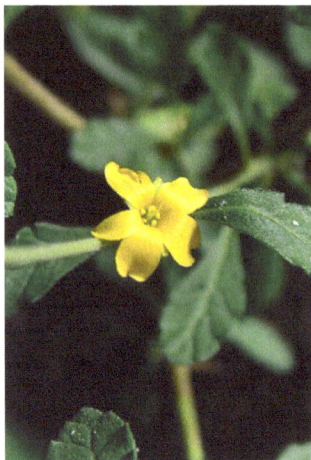

Botanical Classification

Kingdom:	*Plantae*
Order:	*Malpighiales*
Family:	*Passifloraceae*
Genus:	*Turnera*
Species:	*T. Diffusa*

Origin: unknown

Traditional Use:

The entire plant is used to make a tonic.

Uncaria Tomentosa
Common Name: **Cat's claw**

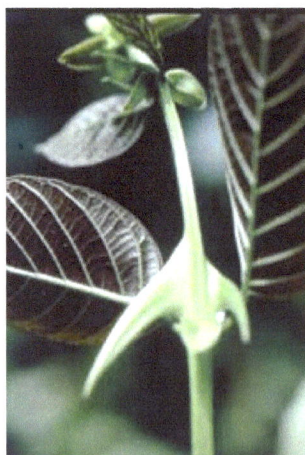

Botanical Classification

Kingdom:	*Plantae*
Order:	*Gentianales*
Family:	*Rubiaceae*
Genus:	*Uncaria*
Species:	*U. Tomentosa*

Origin: South America

Traditional Use:

The leaves of this plant, found in Colombia, Ecuador and Guyana, are used traditionally to treat diabetes.

The leaves are dried and used to make tea.

Zingiber Officinale
Common Name: Ginger

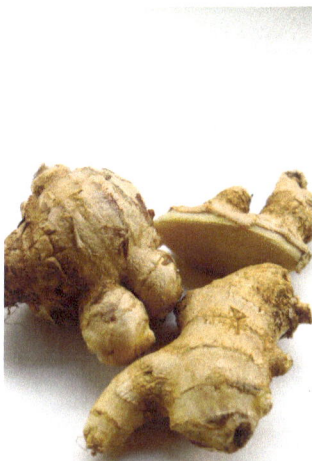

Botanical Classification

Kingdom:	Plantae
Order:	Zingiberales
Family:	Zingiberaceae
Genus:	Zingiber
Species:	Z. Officinale

Origin: West Indies

Traditional Use:

It is used to make ginger tea. It has a therapeutic and protective effect in persons with diabetes. It decreases oxidative stress and hepatic and renal damage.

References:

Ebong, P.E., Eyong, E.U. et al. 2008. 'The Antidiabetic Efficacy of Combined Extracts from Two Continental Plants: Azadirachta indica (A. Juss) (Neem) and Vernonia amygdalina (Del.) (African Bitter Leaf). American Journal of Biochemistry and Biotechnology, no.4:239-244.

Hsu, Y.J., Lee, T.H. et al.2009. 'Anti-hyperglycemic Effects and Mechanism of Bidens pilosa water extract'. Journal of Ethnopharmacology, no.2.

Jain, S., Malviya, S. et al. 2010. 'Antidiabetic Potential of Medicinal Plants; Acta Poloniae Pharmaceutical'. Drug Research, no.2.

Mitra, A. 2006. 'Effects of Fenugreek in Type 2 Diabetes and Dyslipidaemia'. Indian Journal for the Practicing Doctor, no.2.

Olubunmi, A., Adenike, F. et al. 2009. 'Blighia sapida; The Plant and its Hypoglycins An Overview'. Journal of Scientific Research, no. 2.

Palanichamy, S., Nagarajan S. and Devasagayam M. 1988. 'Effect of Cassia alata Leaf Extract on Hyperglycemic Rats'. Journal of Ethnopharmacology, no 22 (1): 81-90

Verma, L., Pawar, R., et al.2010. 'Antidiabetic activity of Cassia occidentalis (Linn) in normal and alloxan-induced diabetic rats'. Indian Journal of Pharmacology, no. 4: 224-228.

5

The Way
Forward

The future of Nutraceuticals is based on innovation through scientific Research and Development (R&D). If this is done appropriately the economic health of countries will certainly be significantly enhanced, particularly developing countries. The major reason for this is because of the significant economic gains which will promote growth and significantly improve gross domestic product (GDP). Therefore, this shift towards embracing science and technology in the direction of the advancement of developing countries is crucial. As such, indigenous produced medicinal plant resources coupled with increased capital investments will result in increased export earnings. This also will stimulate job creation and certainly will enhance the quality of people lives.

However, implementation of these ideas and subsequent injection of capital and resources to achieve economic growth is considerably lacking. Jamaica for example has 84 of the world's 160 major recognized medicinal plants that indigenous to this country. These 84 plants are proven to have tremendous medicinal benefits but are grossly under exploited towards commercialization for wealth creation. Undoubtedly, these ground breaking scientific data resulting from the in-depth analyses of plants with medical properties and proven efficacy, carried out by Caribbean scientist, still only remain published in excellent peer-reviewed scientific journals. To date only two plants from this number have been commercialized either as a formal nutraceutical or as pharmaceutical drug.

It has been stated that a major factor impeding the development of the medicinal plant based industries in developing Caribbean countries for example has been the lack of information on the social and economic benefits that could be derived from the industrial utilization of medicinal plants. Except for the use of these plants for local folklore health care needs, not much information has been available on their market potential and trading possibilities. As a result, the governments and entrepreneurs have not exploited the real potential of these plants.

Therefore, the way forward for Jamaica and the rest of the Caricom region is evidently clear. It is time for the government and the private sector to realize the importance and economic potential of investing in science and technology, for wealth creation where the end result is growth in their respective countries. The translation of these ground breaking scientific findings from indigenous plants must be embraced and aggressively pushed towards the development of novel products either as nutraceuticals or as pharmaceuticals. Overall, the impetus should be geared towards using these plants for the management and or prevention of the vast prevalence of non-communicable diseases; chief among them is diabetes. These important and lucrative nutraceutical and pharmaceutical industries have the potential to spur sustainable livelihoods and entrepreneurial activity in our country's agricultural and health sectors through the provision of value-added products and services, thus facilitating job creation. All this will translate to the overall improvement in health and wellness of the Caribbean people.

Potential Economic Value of plants listed
in Chapter 3

Plants listed in Section II have been identified as ideal candidates for commercial exploitation as drug and or nutraceutical candidates. The scientific evaluations and findings have revealed a strong positive correlation with the reduction in blood glucose levels and improvement in diabetic indices. Therefore, these plants may have tremendous economic potential through commercialization.

It should also be noted that advanced analytical research geared towards the isolation and bioactivity of the isolated molecules, toxicity and clinical testing should be done to assess their safety and efficacy towards the development of a diabetic drug. Additionally, these isolated molecules can be chemically synthesized and modified to produce related products which can be tested for enhanced bioactivity for the treatment and management of the disease.

Importantly, it should be noted that although many of these medicinal plants may show a degree of efficacy in treating symptoms of diabetes (reducing blood sugar levels etc) only a small percentage of these medicinal plants will even produce pharmaceutical drug candidates. A sort of "half way house" with the use of supplements or nutraceuticals is recommended, but should not make specific claims about their efficacy which is a request of most Ministries of Health in relation to nutraceuticals.

Potential Economic Value of plants listed
in Chapter 4

From the plants listed in section III, it is clearly highlighted that these are used extensively in traditional folkloric medicine. However, rigorous scientific analyses have not yet been done on these to determine the efficacy and safety before they can be placed alongside the plants in Section II. On the other hand, although some amount of research has been done to scientifically assess the diabetic potential of some of these plants, the results are far from conclusive and greater amount of research is required. Therefore the use of these plants should be treated with great caution.

Safety of Nutraceuticals and
Pharmaceuticals

The health safety issue of nutraceutical and pharmaceutical products is of paramount importance. Even though plants may exhibit advantageous properties towards the management of or treatment of a particular disease, an extensive toxicological assessment must be thoroughly applied. As such, it should be the responsibility of the researchers and manufacturers to ensure that these products brought to market are safe for consumption and that the consumption of these products will not cause any adverse medical complications.

Legal and Regulatory Framework of the Nutraceutical and Pharmaceutical Industry

The development of Nutraceutical products must be done with great accuracy to ensure the safety and efficacy for persons who will take them. These "drugs" must be manufactured under strict guidelines as set out by the regulations specific for the country in which they are manufactured. For example, in the USA, the Food and Drug Administration (FDA) regulates and set the guidelines for Nutraceutical and Pharmaceutical product development. In Jamaica, the Ministry of Health (MOH) has strict guidelines that must be adhered to (see Jamaica Food and Drug Act, 1975) as it also relates to manufacturing, labelling, importation of these products.

Current regulations that exist by the FDA and by the MOH are designed to cover either foods or drugs - but nothing in between. Not surprisingly, nutraceuticals fall into this gray area between these two categories. However, there is currently no separate system for regulatory compliance only manufacturing guidelines that must be followed. Most of these include general good manufacturing practices (GMP). For example, nutraceuticals must be manufactured in a clean and sterile environment so as to be free of microorganisms and also to ensure that accurate amounts of ingredients are incorporated in to the products. One major regulation for nutraceutical focuses on product labelling which should not provide specific health claims tailored for specific products.

The lack of specific information which addressed the health claims of a nutraceutical product suggests that the regulatory process must be updated to adequately and appropriately address nutraceuticals. The major goal should be to encourage rather than discourage a research-oriented approach to the development and marketing of nutritional products with health benefits. This can be accomplished by creating a regulatory system for nutraceuticals which diminishes the administrative barriers and financial risks for the research and development of important product innovations, and facilitates the development of exclusive and responsible health claims by individual corporations.

Regardless of the form they might take, new regulatory procedures are needed to accommodate the growing array of new products and developments that fall outside the traditional concept of either a food or a drug. In order to be effective and to serve the best interest of the public, this new process should be designed to foster rather than discourage scientific research, encourage the commercial development and availability of important advances, and facilitate the communication of accurate and complete information on nutraceutical products with specific health benefits.

As a result of the widespread use of herbs and nutraceuticals, several international standards have been established in International Pharmacopoeias which have been developed to establish standards for many herbs and related products. These pharmacopoeias include:

- The Ayurvedic Pharmacopoeia of India (API)
- British Herbal Compendium
- British Herbal Pharmacopoeia
- Chinese Herbal Pharmacopoeia
- Japanese Standards for Herbal Medicine
- United States Herbal Pharmacopoeia

Regulation in Jamaica: The Food and Drugs Act

The Jamaican Parliament, in 2000, revised the Food and Drugs Act of 1964 and the food and Drugs Regulations of 1974. The revisions were aimed at ensuring the safety, efficacy, and quality control of herbal products which were approved with the following adaptations:

- Nutraceutical products are subjected to approval,

requirements for which are similar to, but not as elaborate as, those for pharmaceuticals. The onus is on manufacturers to substantiate quality, efficacy and safety of the products.

- Products containing vitamins and minerals in less than three times the recommended daily amount are classified as foods and do not require formal registration.

- Vitamins containing more than three times the recommended amount are classified as drugs.

- Herbal products require registration if they contain substances used for conditions that normally need medical intervention.

- Herbal products containing substances used for self-limiting conditions that do not normally require medical intervention do not require registration.

- Registered products, like drugs, require a permit for importation.

- Products that are not registered do not require a permit for importation; however, proof of quality is required annually or such other time, as deemed necessary.

Conclusion

Unlike traditional herbal remedies, modern or what is referred to as western herbal medicines can be defined as *"a system of medicines which uses various remedies derived from plants such as teas or various plant extracts to maintain health, to treat diseases and other health disorders"*. It is this definition which we need to embrace with the additional note that safety and efficacy need to be realized as far as possible.

In addition to identifying plants which can be exploited for their medicinal value, there is a great need for highly trained professionals who are required to design, develop and administer these alternative remedies. It is therefore noteworthy to highlight that the University of Technology, Jamaica has launched new academic programmes in herbal studies and complementary alternative medicine. This is the first University in the Caribbean region to offer these programmes for which the University of Technology, Jamaica should be commended. This new development will to a great extent support the development of a cadre of qualified personnel who can assist not only with safe practices and quality control, but with the necessary R&D skills to take these ethno-medical practices to the next level. It is hoped that as a result of these developments a "Registry of Consultant Herbalists" as accredited practitioners, can be established to serve not only Jamaica but the entire region.

The demand for herbal therapy is growing exponentially. Herbal medicine which the synthesis of therapeutic experiences of traditional practitioners for hundreds of years particularly for diabetes management is growing significantly in most poor developing countries. Studies have indicated that this growth in popularity is not only because herbal remedies are relatively inexpensive but also because they form better cultural acceptability and better compatibility with the body with minimal side effects. However, recent data indicate that many herbal medicines have some side effects or show little or no efficacy, because there are no defined dosage levels or standards. It is for this reason why *"Herbal Therapy" cannot be used as a substitute for conventional therapy and that herbal remedies should not be viewed as an effective substitute for conventional agents such as oral hypoglycemics and insulin.*

Nevertheless, the years of traditional uses can and often provide us with useful guidelines to the selection, preparation and application of herbal formulation as well as their potential drug development. In order to achieve clinical acceptance vigorous methods of scientific and clinical validation need to be applied to prove their safety and efficacy.

Currently 80% of the world population depends on plant-derived medicine for the first line of primary health care for human alleviation because these herbals have minimal side effects. It should be noted that plants are important sources of medicines and presently about 25% of all pharmaceutical prescriptions in the United States contain at least one plant-derived ingredient. In the last century, roughly 121 pharmaceutical products were formulated based on the traditional knowledge obtained from various sources.

Medicinal plants have and will continue to play an important role in the development of potent therapeutic agents. It should be noted that from 1950-1970 approximately 100 new plant-based new drugs were developed in the USA. These include for example, Reserpine, Vinblastine and Vincristine. From 1971 to 1990 new drugs such as Nabiloine, Aartemisinin and Ginkgolides were developed. Of all the new drugs introduced from 1991 to 1995 (2%) including Pacilaxel and Toptecan were from plant sources.

Future Prospects of Herbal Medicine Market

It is estimated that nearly three fourths of the herbal drugs used worldwide were discovered following leads from local medicine. According to WHO about 25% of modern medicines have been developed from traditional medicinal plants. Several other drugs which are synthetic analogues have built on prototype compounds isolated from plants. Based on these observations and the vast potential which exists for the exploitation of medicinal plants for pharmaceuticals and nutraceuticals, a case can be made for further R&D work for the development and commercialization of these vital natural product resources.

Annex

Ten Rules for Collecting Medicinal Plants

1. Equip yourself with good, precise knowledge of the medicinal plant

2. Poisonous/dangerous plants and ones that they resemble should not be gathered by children

3. If plants are to be collected for sale, it is best to specialize in collecting one particular specie

4. Never gather all specimens when collecting in the wild; leave some for its continued survival

5. Always wear gloves when collecting plants, and use tools such as knives and sickles

6. Select the proper receptacle for the parts of the plants to be collected, and store loosely

7. Gather only healthy, visibly undamaged plants (not infested with pests or diseases)

8. Do not gather medicinal plants in grasslands where pesticides and weed killers are used

9. Plants should not be gathered when they are wet with rain/dew, as this can reduce concentration of their active constituents

10. After harvesting, collected plants should be dried, aerated and stored in suitable containers in a dry, dark place at low temperatures (below15°C)

Storing Drugs

The generally accepted principle is that long storage reduces the efficacy of a drug, as overtime, its bioactive constituents break down. Accordingly, it is recommended that drugs over two years old should not be used, and to replace drugs for their use yearly. Additionally, proper storage is paramount to preserving the potency of a drug. Large quantities of drugs can be stored in burlap sacks, cartons, drums and metal containers. (Plastic containers should not be used). Stored drugs should be discarded if they become infested with pests.

Labelling Stored Drugs

All stored drugs should be properly and carefully labelled, ensuring that the label also contains the year the drug was harvested. Poisonous drugs should be marked with the warning symbol ☠.

Resources for Suggested Reading

Research Guidelines for Evaluating The Safety and Efficacy of Herbal Medicines
WHO Regional Office for the Western Pacific – 1993

Basic Tests for Drugs: Pharmaceutical Substances, Medicinal Plant Materials and Dosage Forms
1998

Basic Tests for Pharmaceutical Dosage Forms
1991

Basic Tests for Pharmaceutical Substances
1986

The International Pharmacopoeia, their edition
Volume 1: General Methods Of Analysis – *1979*
Volume 2: Quality Specifications - 1981
Volume 3: Quality Specifications – *1988*

Volume 4: Tests, Methods, and General Requirements; Quality

Specifications for Pharmaceutical Substances,
Excipients and Dosage Forms.
1994

Jamaica Food and Drug Act, 194 and 1975

**Quality Assurance of Pharmaceuticals: A Compendium of
Guidelines and Related Materials,** *Vol. 1*
1997

**WHO Expert Committee on Specifications for
Pharmaceutical Preparations**
*Thirty-fourth repor*t
WHO Technical Report Series, No 863
1996

Glossary

Anti-Hyperglycemic Agents

An antibody produced by the body's immune system that is directed at one or more of the individual's own proteins. Autoimmune responses typically lead to a wide array of medical conditions such as Type I diabetes, rheumatoid arthritis and lupus erythematosus.

Auto-Antibodies:

An antibody produced by the body's immune system that is directed at one or more of the individual's own proteins. Autoimmune responses typically lead to a wide array of medical conditions such as Type I diabetes, rheumatoid arthritis and lupus erythematosus.

Beta Cells

Highly specialized cells found in the islets of Langerhans in the pancreas that produce and secrete insulin into the bloodstream.

Bioactive

Biological substance that interacts with or has an effect on any cell or tissue in the body.

Cerebrovascular

Pertaining to the blood vessels especially the arteries that supply the brain.

Diabetic Ketoacidosis

Is a problem that occurs in people with diabetes. It occurs when the body cannot use sugar (glucose) as a fuel source because there is no insulin or not enough insulin. Fat is used for fuel instead and when broken down are called ketones, that build up in the blood and urine.

These ketones are poisonous and the condition is known as ketoacidosis.

Dosage	Quantity of medicine or substance prescribed or administered to an organism.
Drugs	A chemical substance used in the treatment, cure, prevention, or diagnosis of diseases or used to otherwise enhance physical or mental well-being.
Ethnomedicine	Study of traditional medicines with both substantiated and unsubstantiated health claims.
Etiology	The causes or origin of a disease.
Exocrine	Secreting to an epithelial surface.
Extracts	A solution or mixture containing the active principles of a drug or plant.
Folklore	A body of widely held unsubstantiated claims.
Glucose	A simple sugar (carbohydrate, monosaccharide) obtained from digested food and used a source of energy in the body.
HbA1 C	A diagnostic test that detects how much glucose has been present in the bloodstream over the last 2 to 3 months. It is also referred to as A1C, Hemoglobin A1C, and glycohemoglobin testing.
Hypercholesterolemia	The is the presence of high levels of cholesterol in the blood.

Hyperglycemia	Commonly referred to as high blood sugar, is a condition in which an excessive amount of glucose circulates in the blood.
Hyperlipidemia	A condition of abnormally elevated levels of any or all lipids and/or lipoproteins in the blood.
Hypertrophy	Enlargement of an organ or part thereof resulting from an increase in the size of the cells.
Hypoglycemia	Commonly referred to as low blood sugar, is a condition in which there are abnormally. low levels of glucose in the blood.
Insulin	Hormone produced by the pancreas that is essential in regulating carbohydrate and fat metabolism in the body.
Insulinopathy	A monogenic form of adult-onset diabetes due to mutations in the insulin gene.
Myocardial Infarction	A heart attack that results in the irreversible death of heart muscle from the sudden blockage of a coronary artery by a blood clot.
Nephropathy	Refers to damage to or disease of the kidney.
Neuropathy	A collection of disorders that occurs when nerves of the peripheral nervous system (the part of the nervous system outside of the brain and spinal cord) are damaged.
Nutraceutical	A food or food product that reportedly provides health and medical benefits, including the. prevention and treatment of disease.

Oxidative Stress	A condition of increased oxidant production in animal cells characterize by the release of free radicals and resulting in cellular degeneration.
Pancreatopathy	Disease of the pancreas.
Pathophysiology	The study of the changes of normal mechanical, physical and biochemical functions, either caused by a disease, or resulting from an abnormal syndrome.
Pharmaceutical	A chemical substance intended for use in the medical diagnosis, cure, treatment, or prevention of disease.
Retinopathy	Any diseased condition of the retina in the eye, especially one that is non-inflammatory.
Type 2 Diabetes Mellitus	A metabolic disorder that is characterized by high blood glucose in the context of insulin resistance and relative insulin deficiency.
Type I Diabetes Mellitus	A form of diabetes mellitus that results from autoimmune destruction of insulin-producing beta cells of the pancreas. The subsequent lack of insulin leads to increased blood and urine glucose.

About the Authors

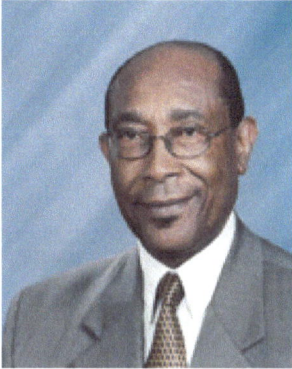

HENRY I. C. LOWE
C.D., J.P., Ph.D., F.R.S.H., A.R.I.C

Dr. Henry Lowe is a scientist who specializes in medicinal chemistry and has contributed over 40 years in the fields of science and technology, energy, the environment, wellness and health sciences nationally, regionally and internationally. Dr. Lowe is not only recognized as one of the regions outstanding scientists but also public servant, author, educator and successful entrepreneur. He has co-authored numerous publications related to science, education, environment, and health. Dr. Lowe is a past Chairman of the Bureau of Standards Jamaica and the Scientific Research Council. In addition, he is the past President & CEO of the former Blue Cross of Jamaica, and also served as its Chairman. Dr. Lowe is the Founder/Executive Chairman of the Environmental Health Foundation, Owner of Eden Gardens Wellness & Lifestyle Centre and also the Founder/Chairman of Bio-Tech R&D Institute Ltd., Jamaica. He is the newly appointed Deputy Chairman for the Scientific Research Council.

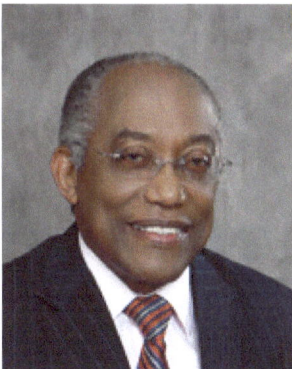

ERROL ST. A. Y. MORRISON
OJ, MD, PhD, FRCP (Glasg), FACP, FRSM (UK), FRSH (UK), FJIM

Professor the Honourable Errol Morrison has had a long and distinguished career in medicine, academia and the voluntary social services. In 1992, he was appointed Professor of Biochemistry and in 1994, Professor of Endocrinology by the University of the West Indies (UWI). In 1999, he was made Pro Vice Chancellor and Dean, School for Graduate Studies & Research, UWI. In 1993, Professor Morrison founded the University Diabetes Outreach Programme (UDOP), which now hosts the largest annual international diabetes conference in the Caribbean region. Since 2007, UDOP spearheads and coordinates diabetes related activities at the University of the West Indies (UWI), the University of Technology, Jamaica (UTech) and Northern Caribbean University (NCU). Professor Morrison is the President of the University of Technology, Jamaica and Life President of the Diabetes Association of Jamaica.

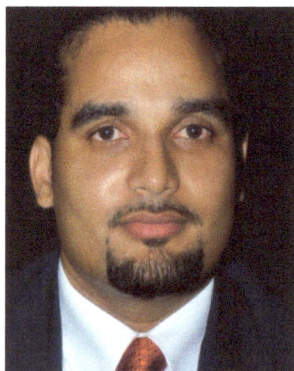

PERCEVAL S. BAHADO-SINGH
Ph.D

Dr. Perceval Bahado-Singh is the Director of Research and Development at the Bio-Tech R&D Institute. He has served as a Research Scientist at the Scientific Research Council of Jamaica and as a Research Fellow at the University of the West Indies, Faculty of Medical Sciences. He holds a PhD in Biotechnology and a BSc (Hons) double major in Biochemistry and Zoology from the University of the West Indies, Mona. He has authored several books and his peer-reviewed publications focus on diabetes, biochemical evaluation and mechanism of action of drugs of abuse (cocaine and marijuana), nutrition and bioactive molecules from medicinal plants for the treatment of prostate cancer. Dr. Bahado-Singh is currently a reviewer for several peer-reviewed journals which centers on his current scientific interests including the treatment and management of type 2 diabetes; stem cell research; natural products and nutraceutical development.

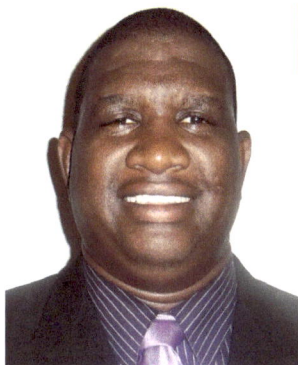

CLIFF K. RILEY
Ph.D

Dr. Cliff Riley is an Associate Professor and Associate Dean of Graduate Studies and Research in the College of Health Sciences, University of Technology, Jamaica. He holds a PhD in Biotechnology (Pharmaceutical) and a Bachelor of Science Degree in Chemistry and Biochemistry from the University of the West Indies, Mona. Dr. Riley has served as Research Scientist at the Scientific Research Council, Associate Director of Research at the Northern Caribbean University and Coordinator for Graduate Studies and Research at the College of Health Sciences, UTech, Jamaica. Dr. Riley has done extensive research and published numerous scientific papers in diabetes management and education, nutrition, food technology, pharmaceutics and natural products. He is an active member of several professional organizations including the Biochemical Society, UK, Carnegie Foundation for Cancer Research, the Caribbean Academy of Science and board member of the Diabetes Association of Jamaica